Exercises in Radiological Diagnosis

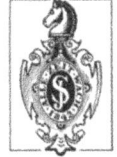

A. Wackenheim   A. Badoz

Computed Tomography
of the Abdomen in Adults

85 Radiological Exercises for Students and
Practitioners

With 357 Illustrations

Springer-Verlag
Berlin Heidelberg New York
London Paris Tokyo

Professor Dr. Auguste Wackenheim
Hospices Civils de Strasbourg
Centre Hospitalier Régional
Service de Radiologie 1
1, Place de l'Hôpital
F-67091 Strasbourg Cedex

Dr. Armelle Badoz
Centre de Traumatologie et d'Orthopédie
10, Avenue Baumann
F-67400 Illkirch-Graffenstaden

Translated from the French by
Marie-Thérèse Wackenheim

Library of Congress Cataloging-in-Publication Data. Wackenheim, A. (Auguste) Computed tomography of the abdomen in adults. (Exercises in radiological diagnosis) Translation of: Tomodensitométrie de l'adulte. Includes index. 1. Abdomen–Diseases–Diagnosis–Problems, exercises, etc. 2. Tomography–Problems, exercises, etc. I. Badoz, A. (Armelle), 1952- . II. Title. III. Series. RC944.W3213 1988 617'.5507572 88-1981

ISBN-13: 978-3-540-16540-8 e-ISBN-13: 978-3-642-71192-3
DOI: 10.1007/978-3-642-71192-3

2127/3130-543210 – Printed on acid-free paper

Contents

Introduction

These exercises are meant for students and practitioners who wish to familiarize themselves with the normal and pathological computerized tomographic radioanatomy of the abdomen.

The iconography is sufficiently characteristic to be read without the help of clinical or biological data. It comprises both normal and pathologic findings.

Analysis of scans is comprised of two steps. The first part consists of the detailed study of normal scans, which serve as a reference. For this, eight main slice levels have been considered necessary and sufficient: necessary since a certain number of slices are indispensable for the exploration of the abdomen; sufficient because a larger number of slices would risk rendering memorization difficult. The second part involves a study of the pathologic findings, organ by organ.

Acknowledgements. Appreciation is extended to all those who have helped in realizing this study and, more particularly, to our friends and colleagues, J. L. DIETEMANN, C. ROY, J. L. BURGUET, M. VOUGE, and J. W. SOUTTER.

We would also like to thank Dr. J. WIECZOREK for his friendly assistance and advice in the planning and presentation of figures and schemata.

1

Technical Note

Computerized tomography of the abdomen begins with an initial image called "scout view". This numbered radiograph of the abdomen is an analogous representation of the information and allows the location of the eight selected slice levels; these are represented by horizontal lines. The slices are 10 mm thick and are taken at intervals of 2.5 cm.

Schemata and corresponding text are found in Part 2. These utilize numbers which correspond either to the reference slice or to references in the text.

Note also that the hollow organs of the digestive tract are hachured on the schemata.

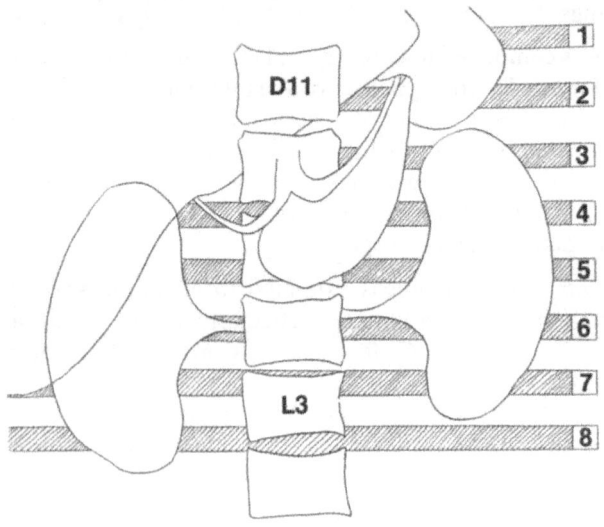

Part One

Iconography

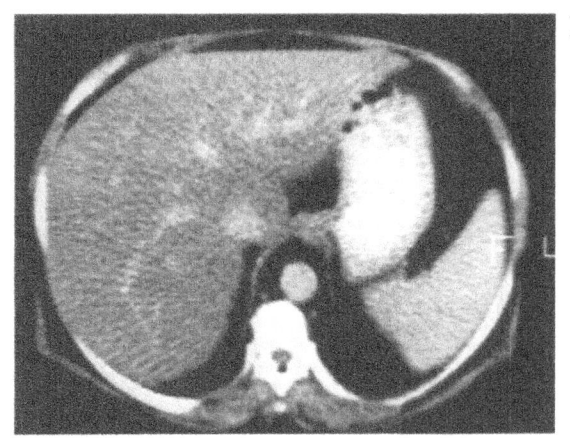

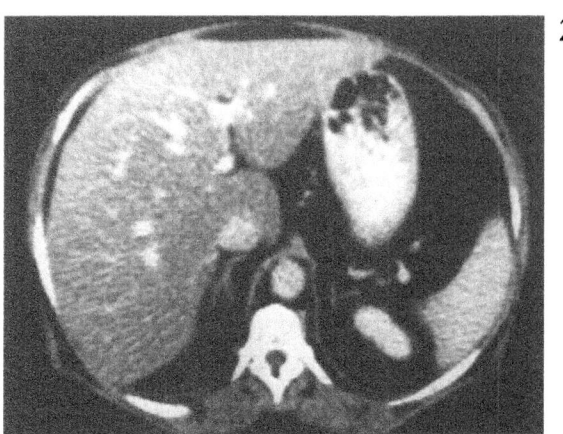

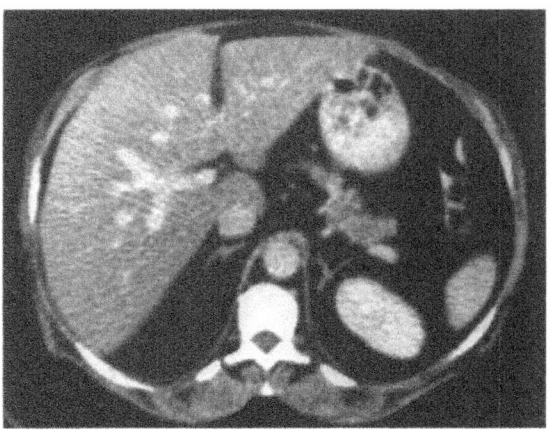

4

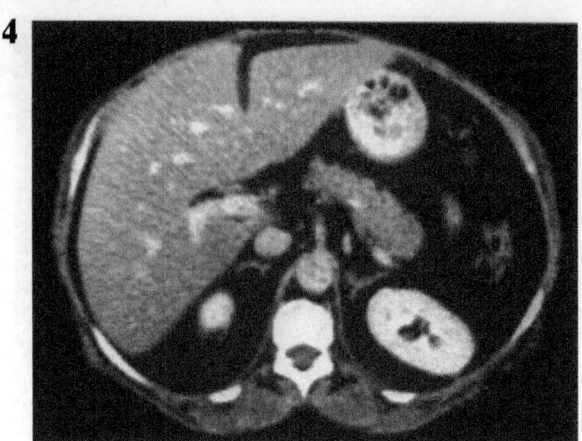

5

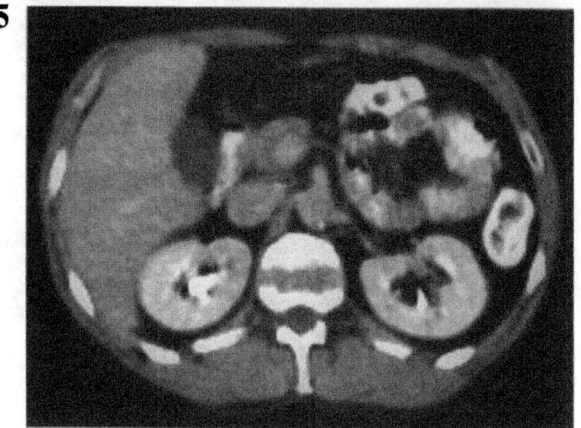

6

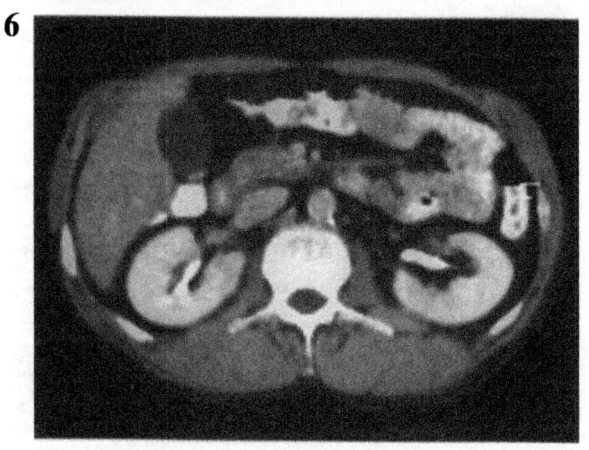

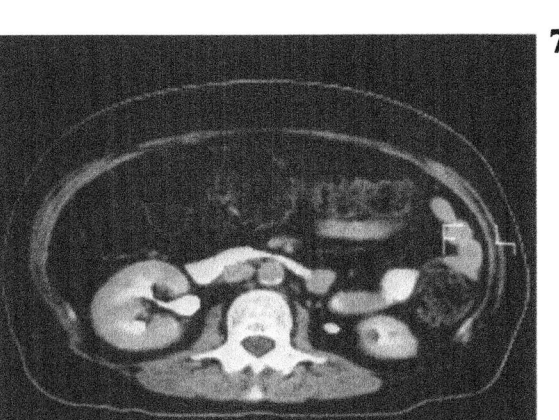

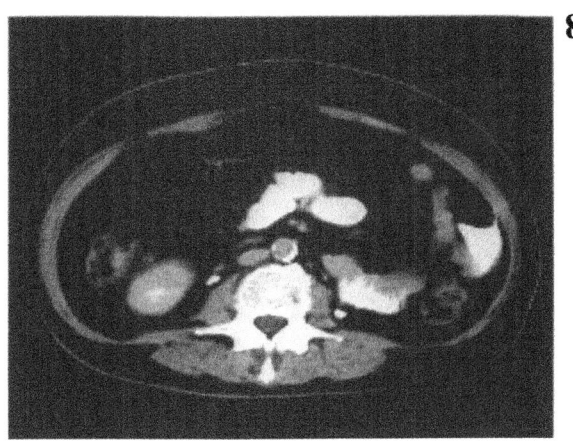

9

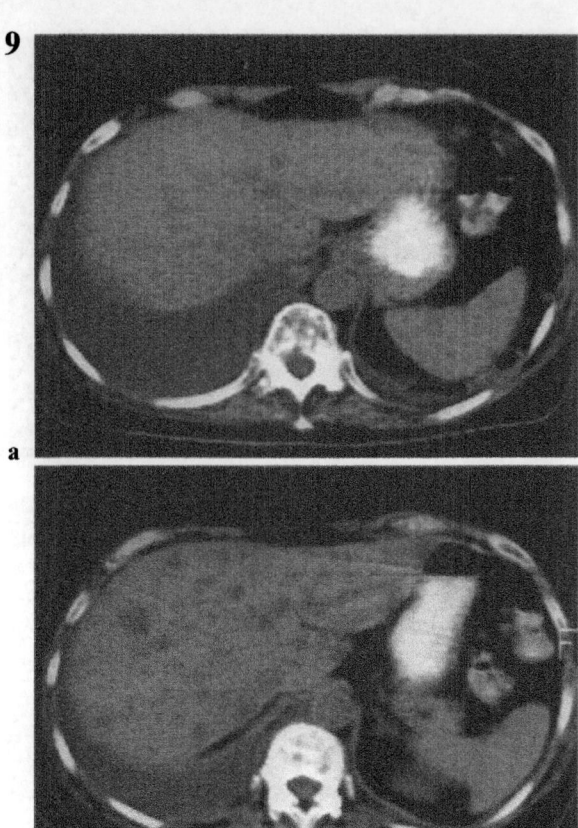

a

c

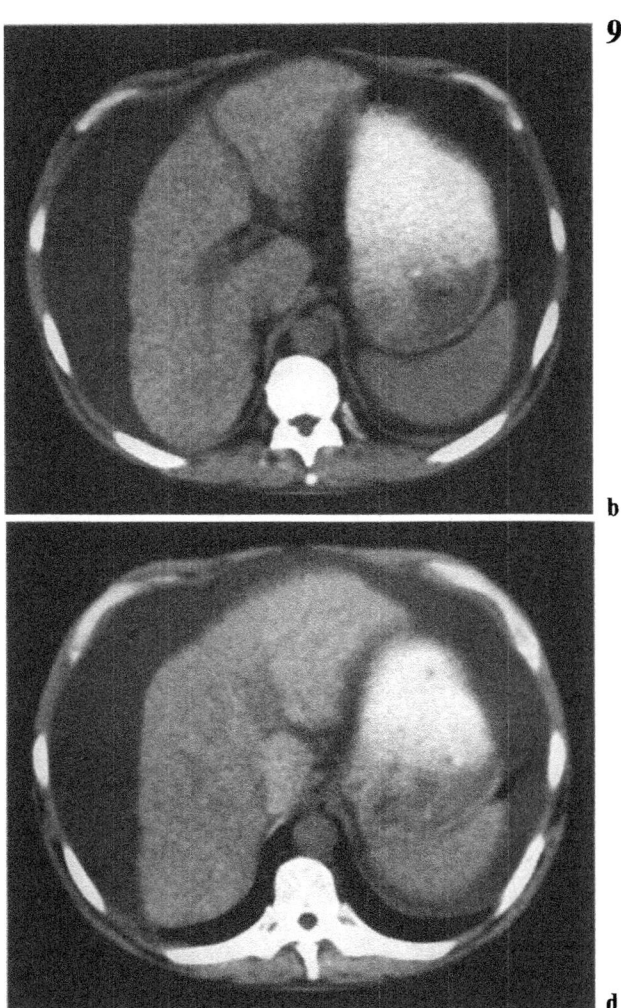

9

b

d

10

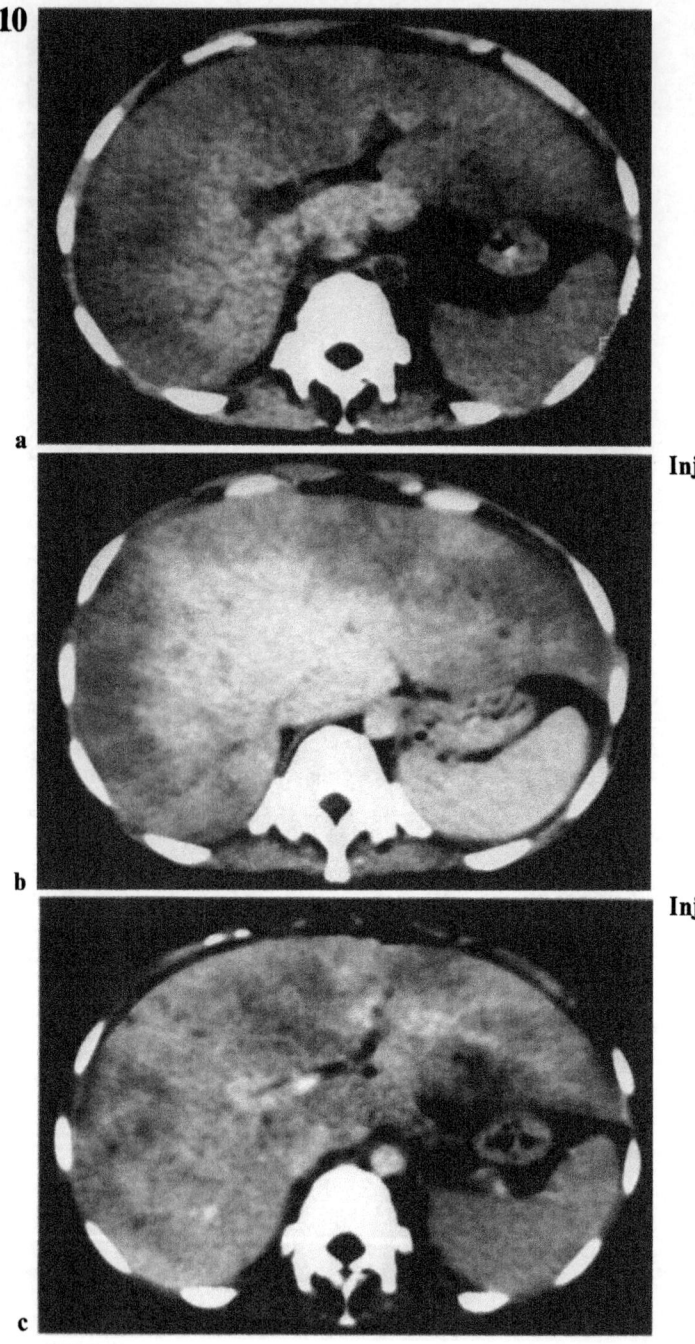

a

Inj.

b

Inj.

c

Inj. **11**

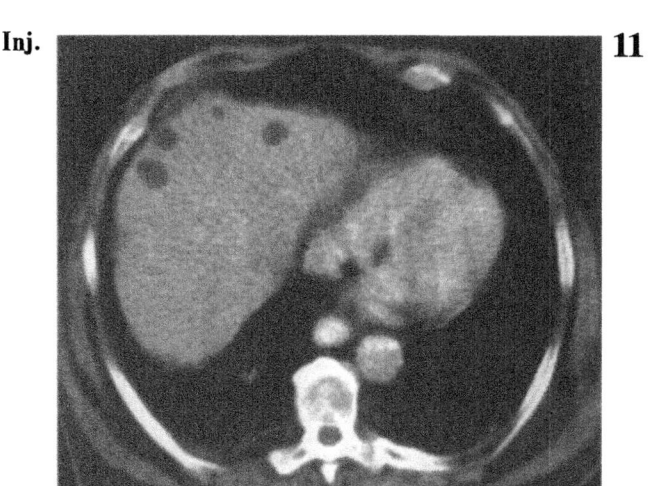

Inj. **12**

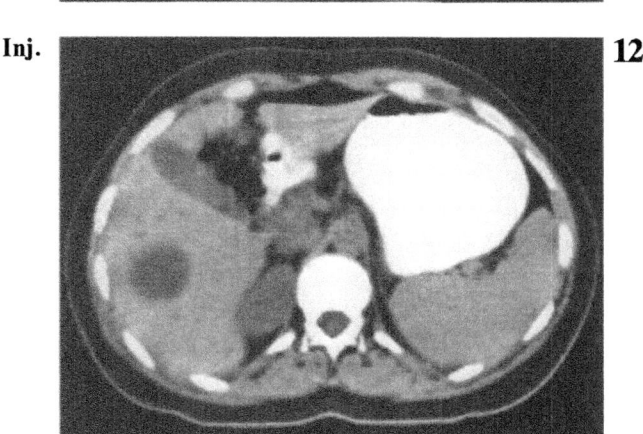

Inj. **13**

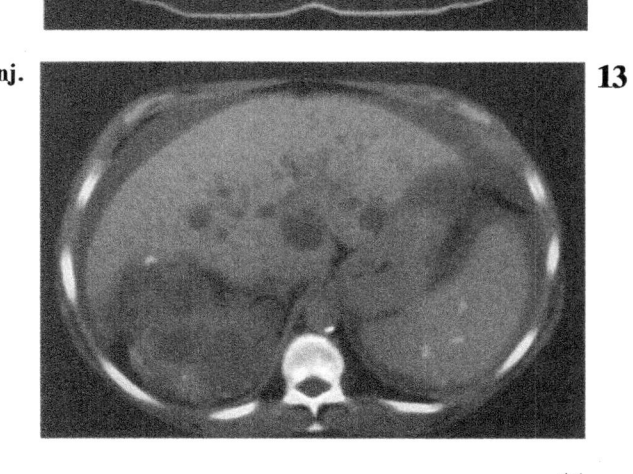

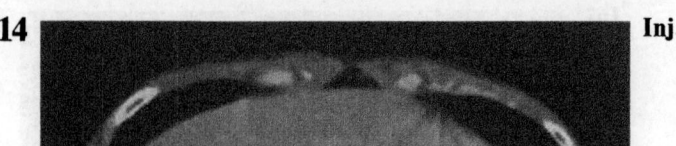

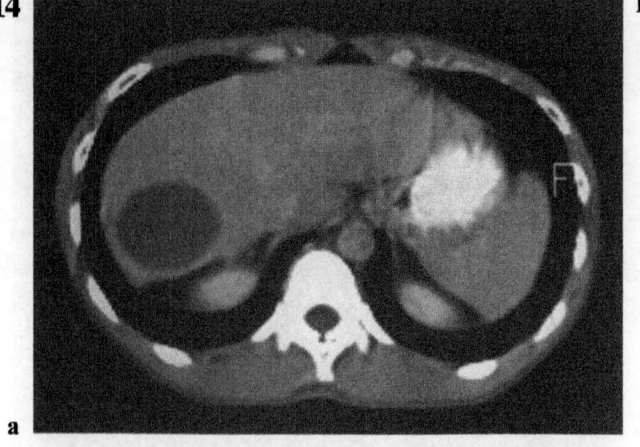

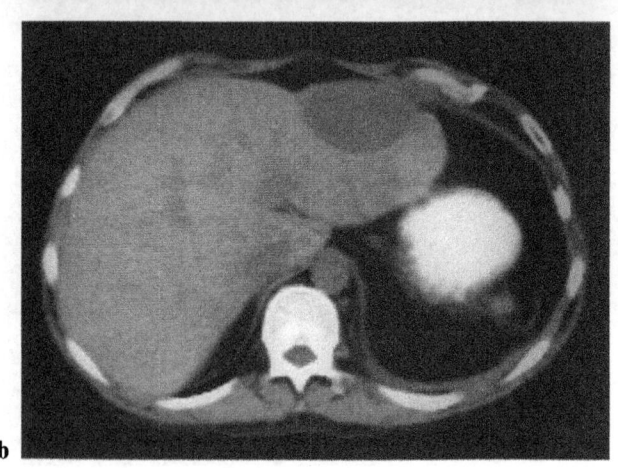

Inj.

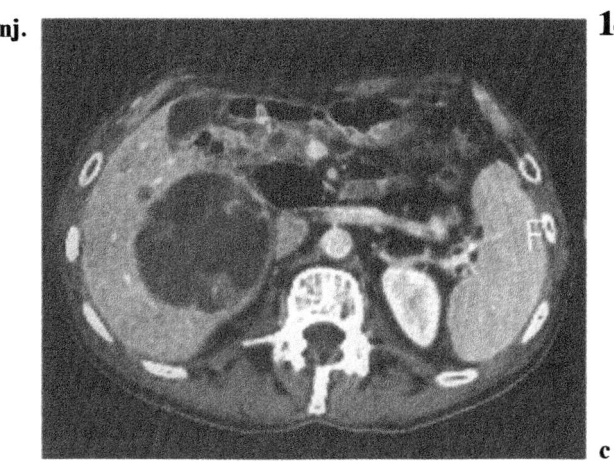

c

Inj.

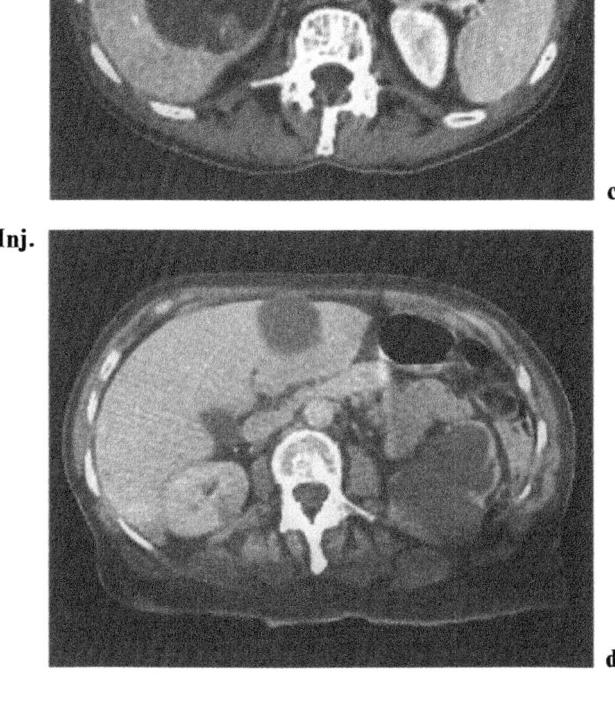

d

15

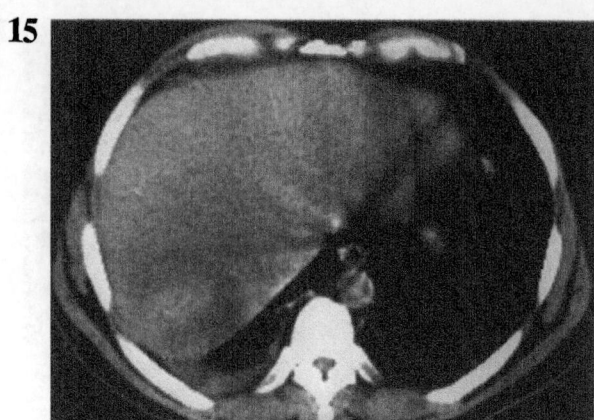

16

Inj.

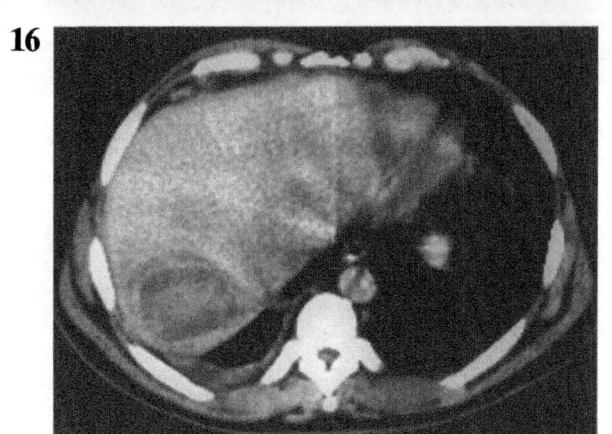

17

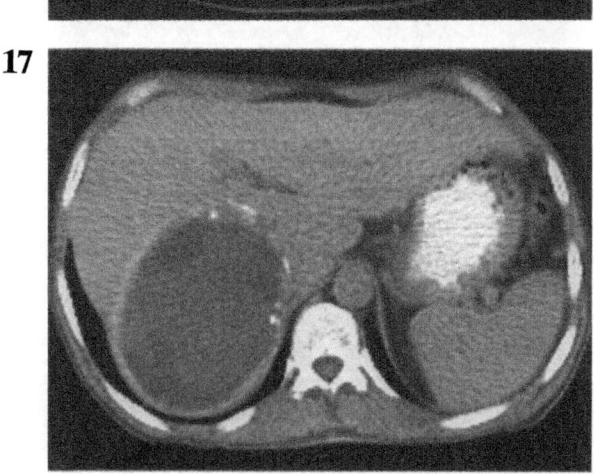

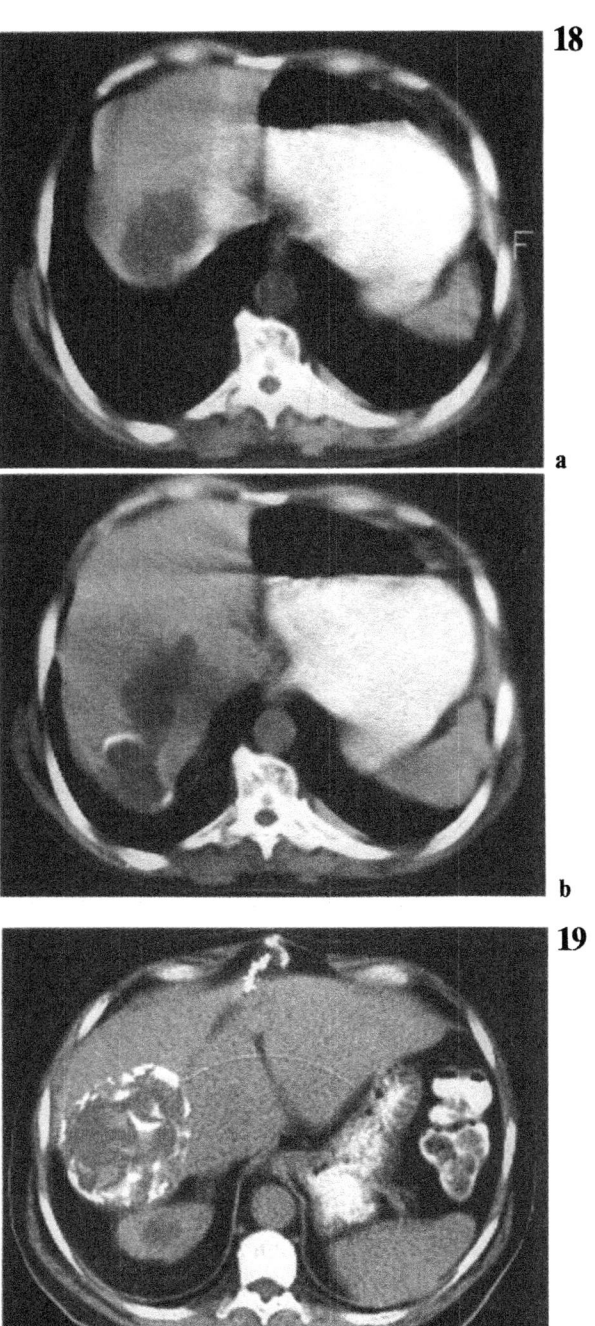

a

b

20

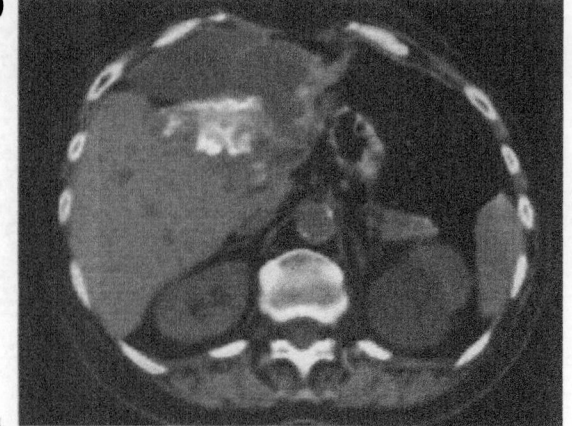

Inj.

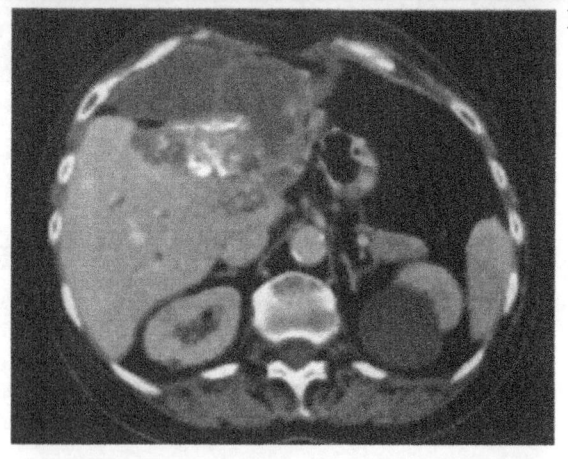

21

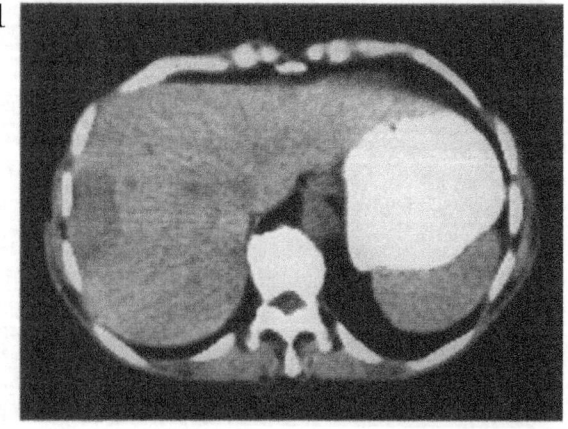

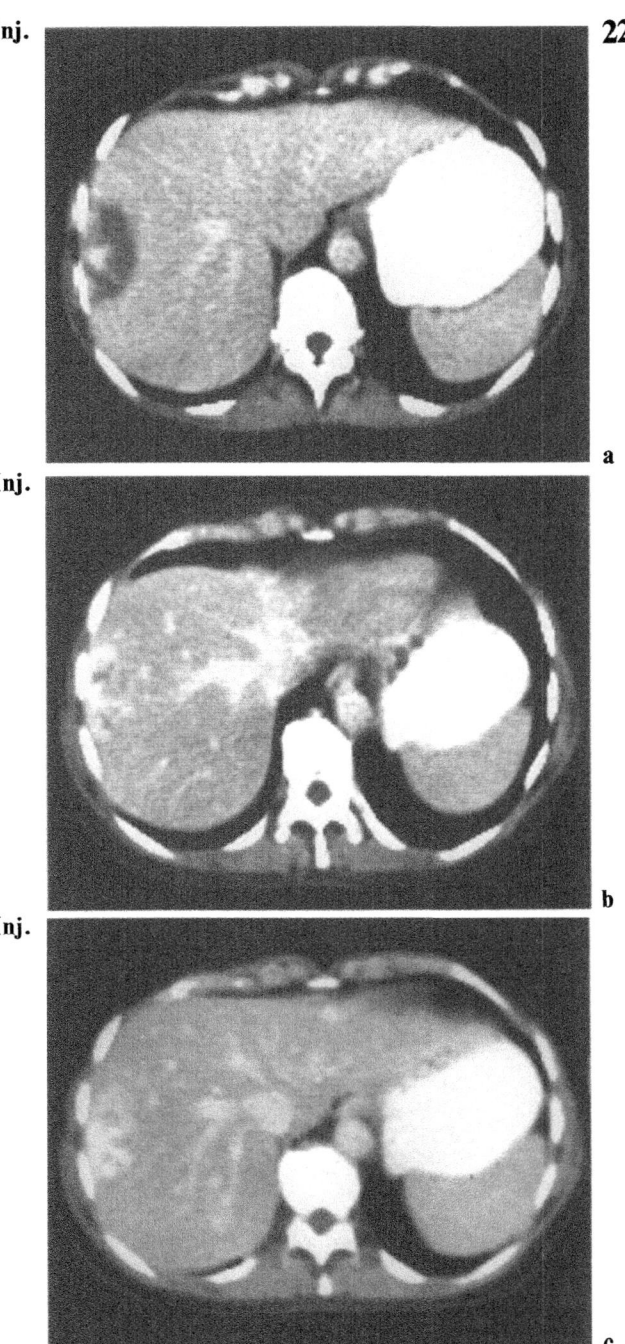

23

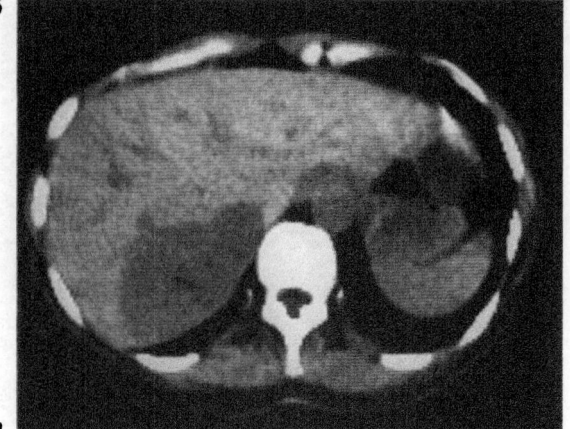

Inj.

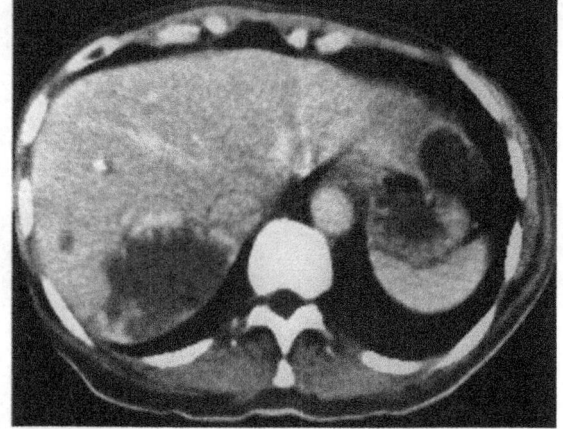

Inj.

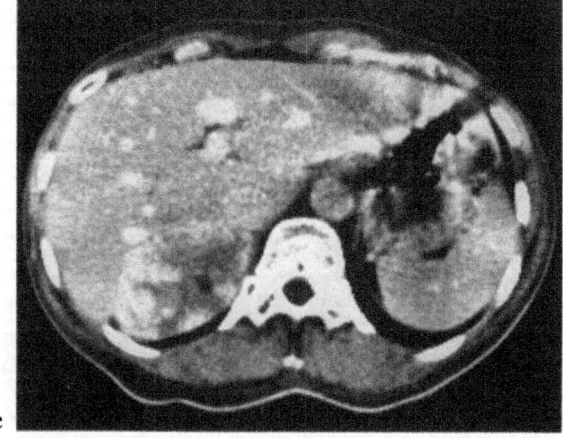

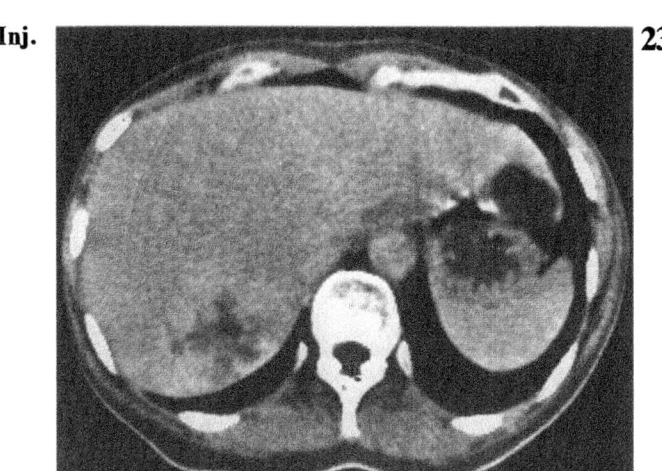

d

24

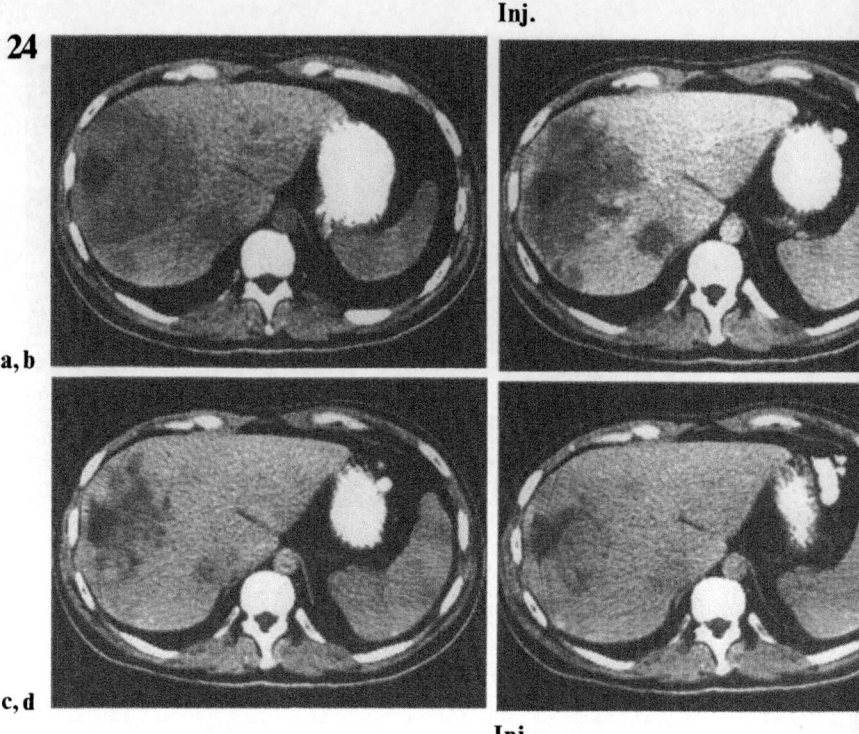

a, b

c, d

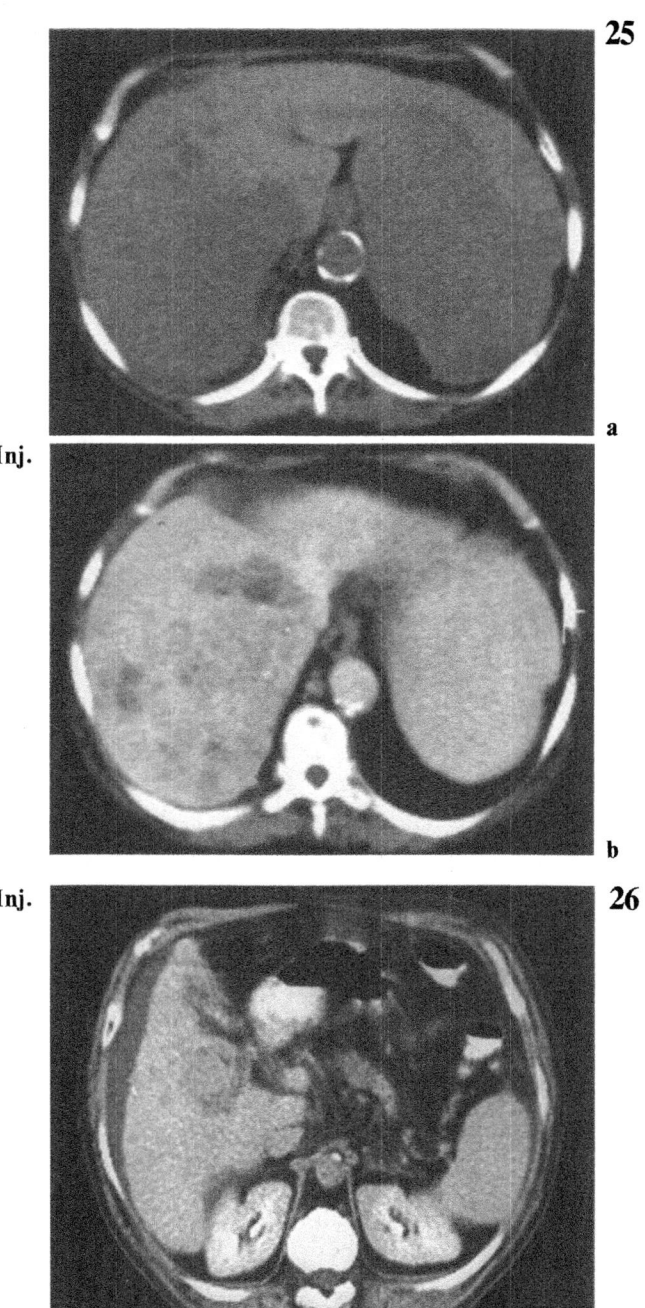

25

Inj.

b

Inj. **26**

a

26

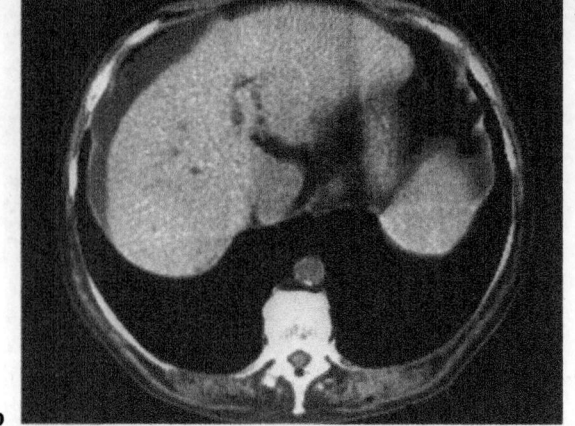

b

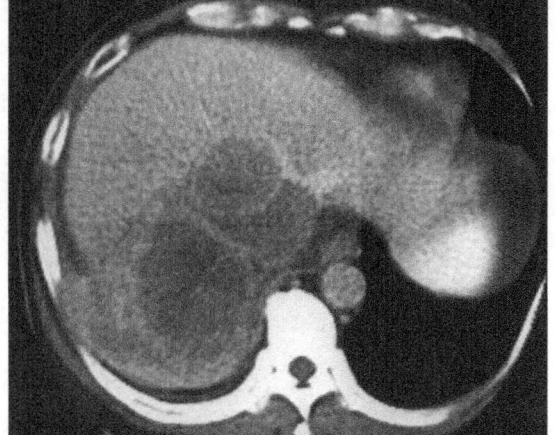

c

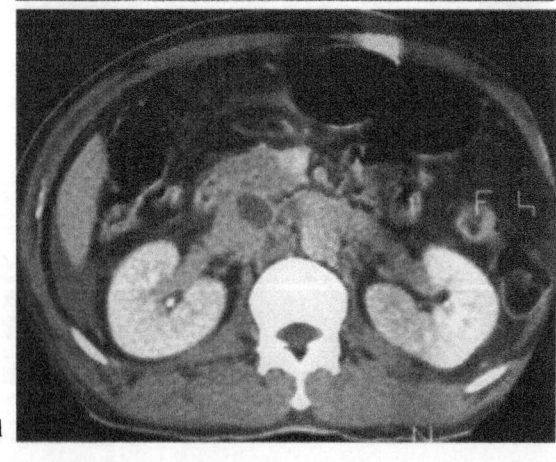

d

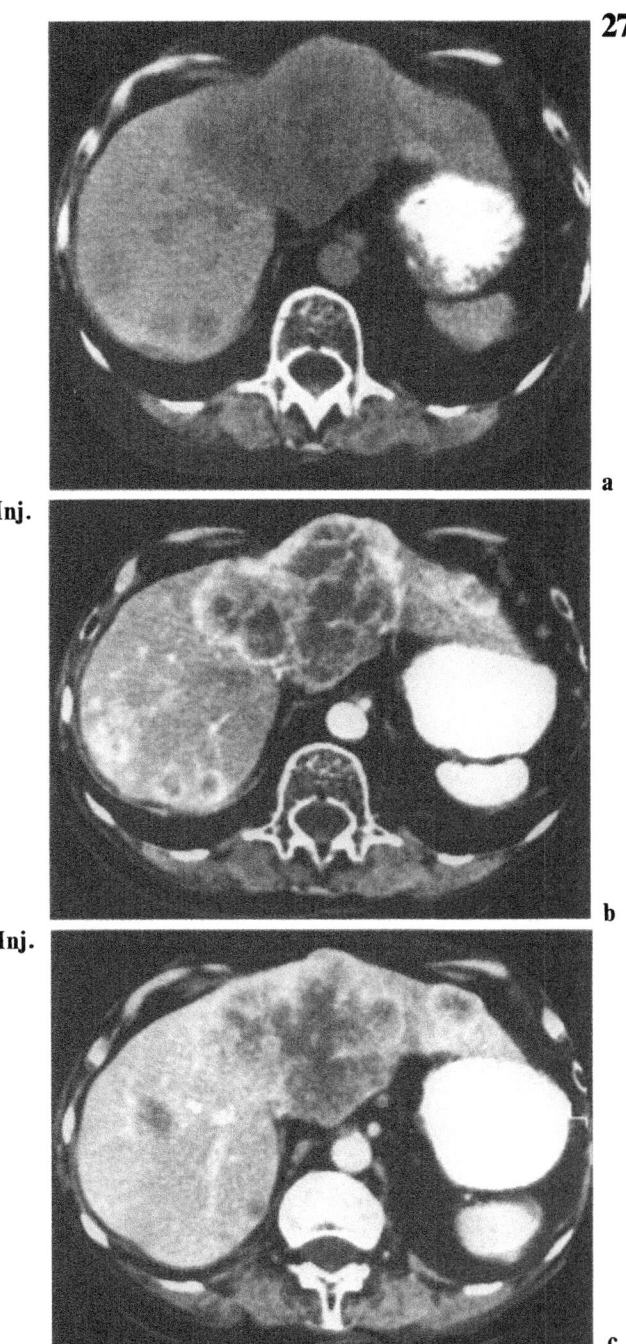

Inj.

Inj.

a

b

c

28   Inj.

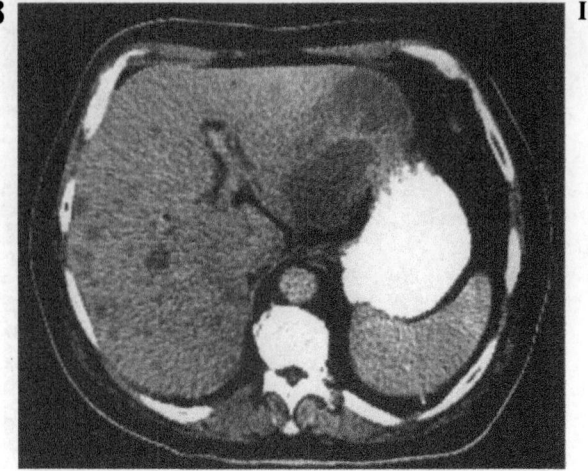

29   Inj.

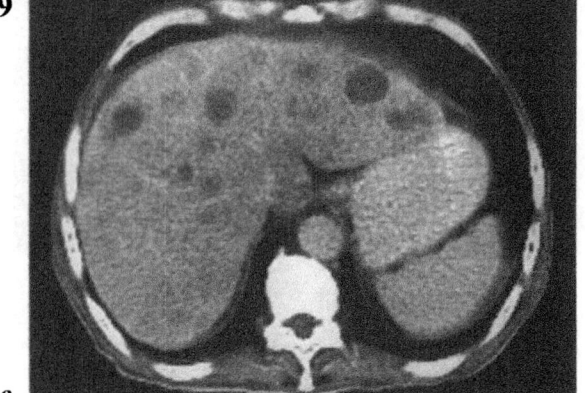

a

                                              Inj.

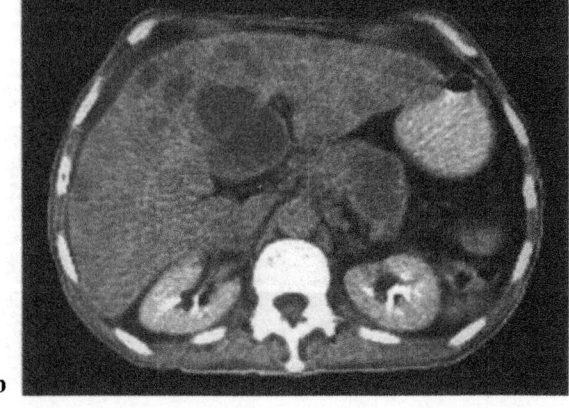

b

24

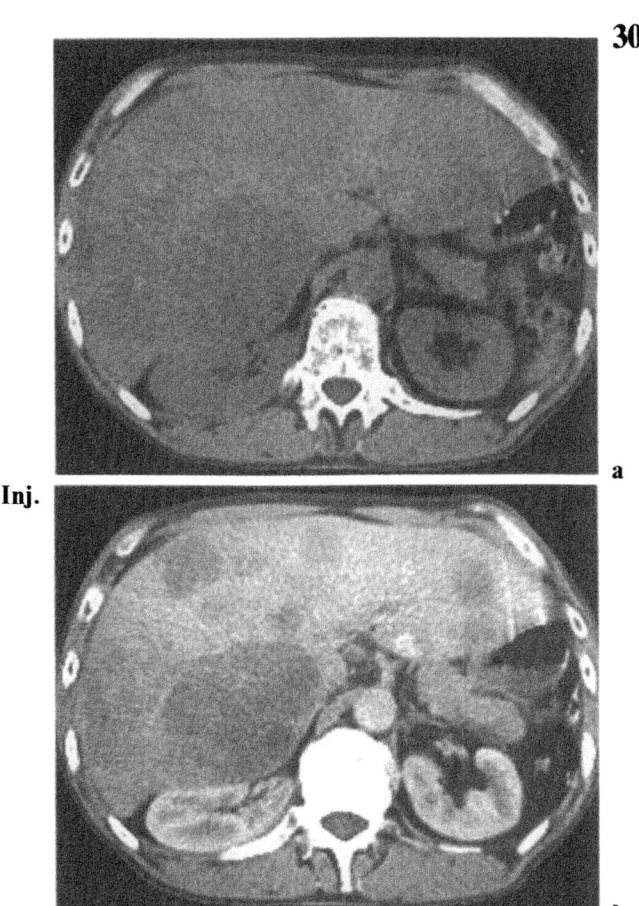

Inj.

a

b

30

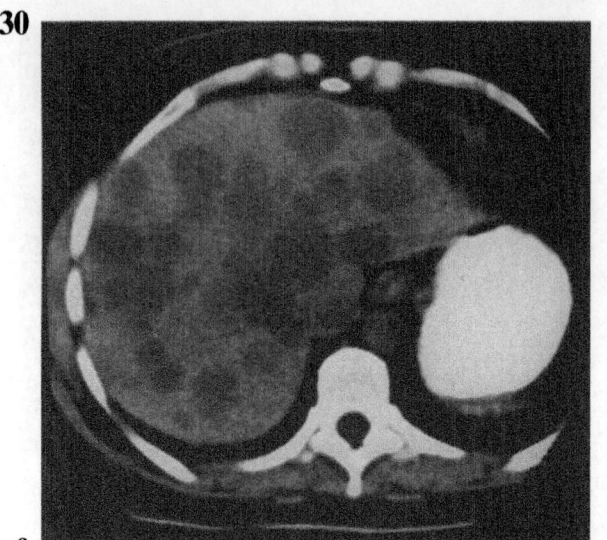

c

Inj.

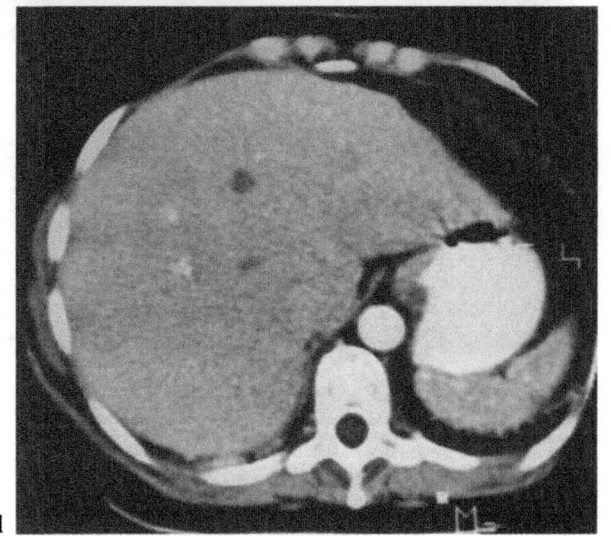

d

31

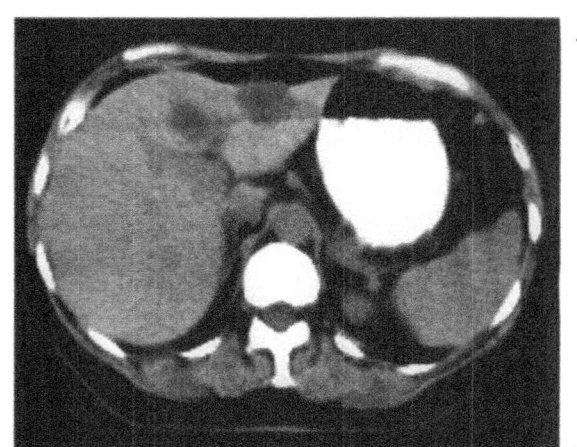

Inj.

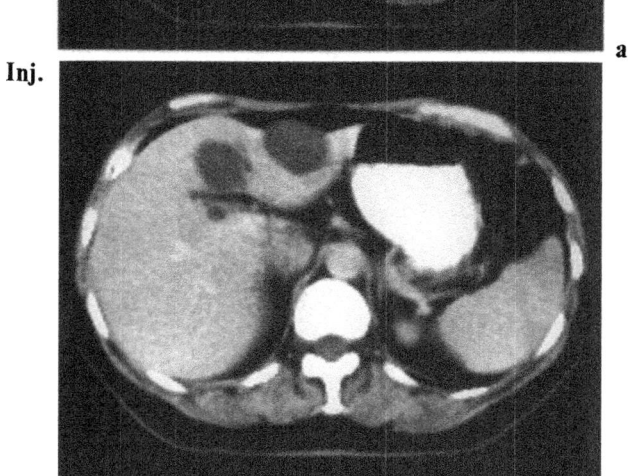

a

b

27

32

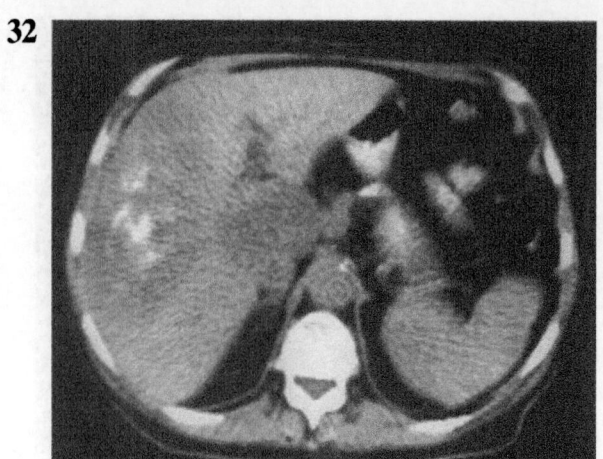

a

Inj.

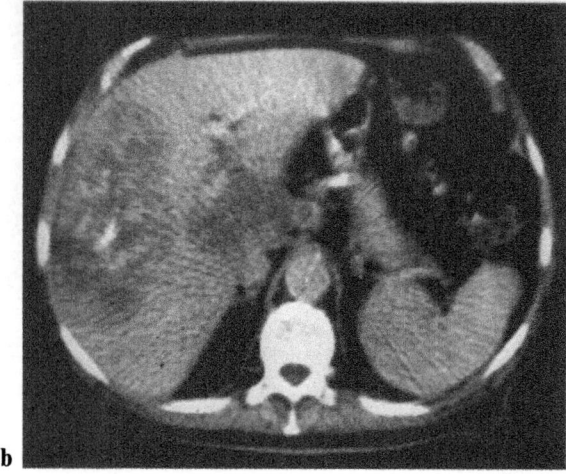

b

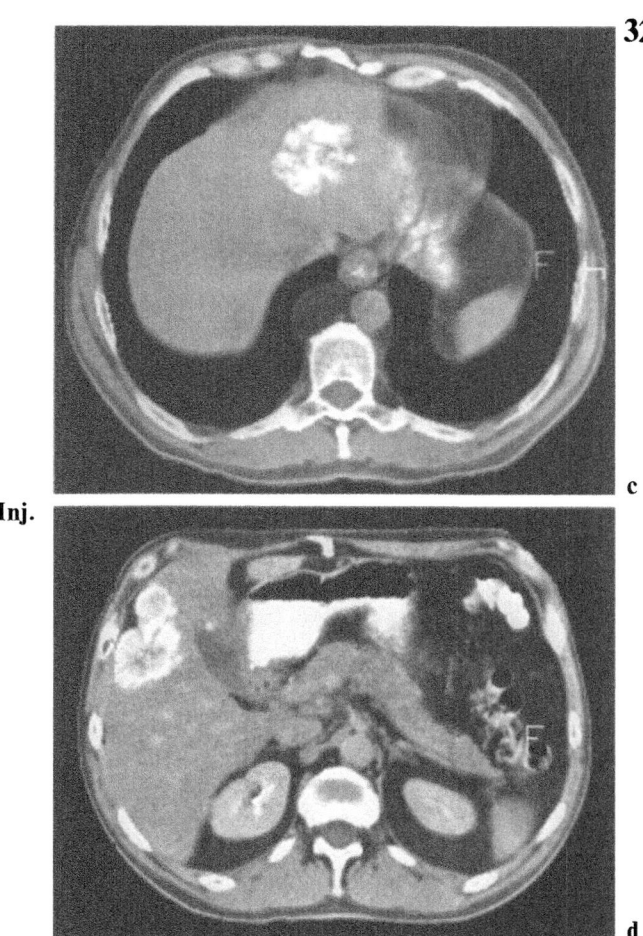

Inj.

c

d

33

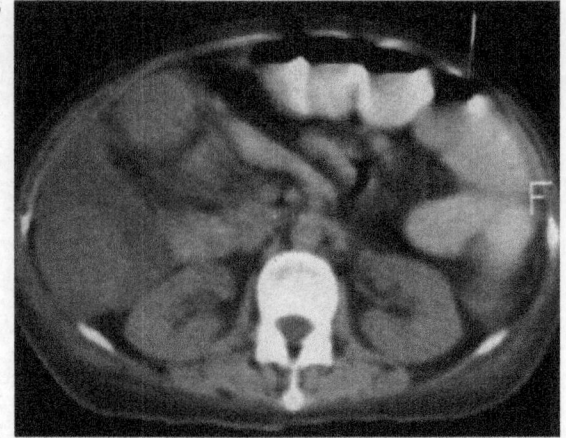

Inj.

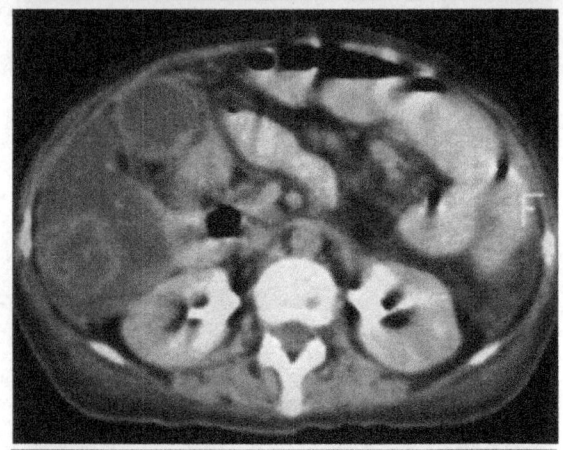

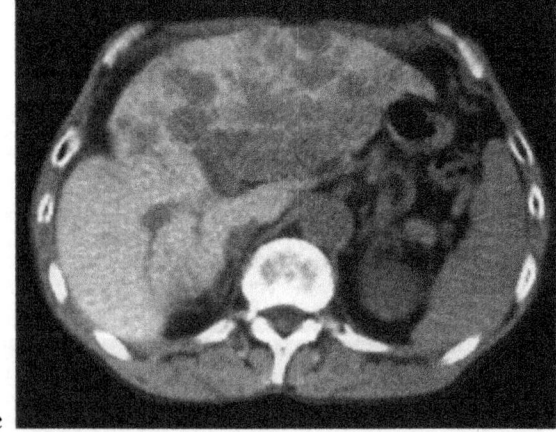

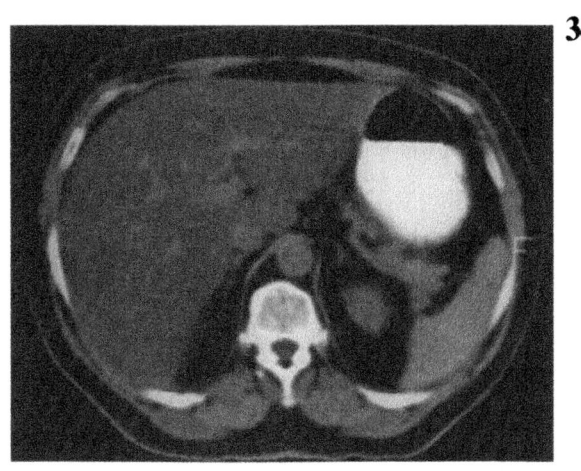

34

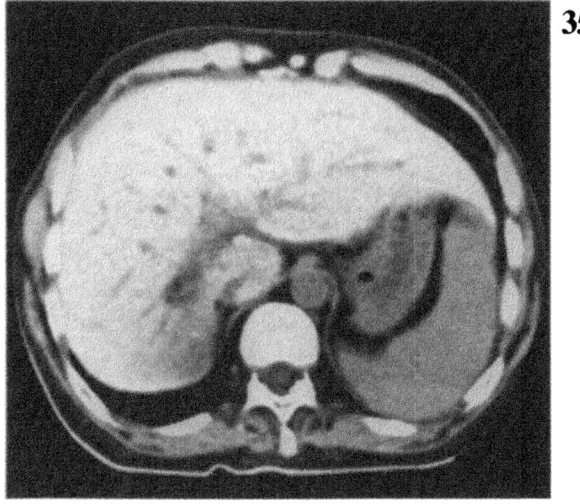

35

36

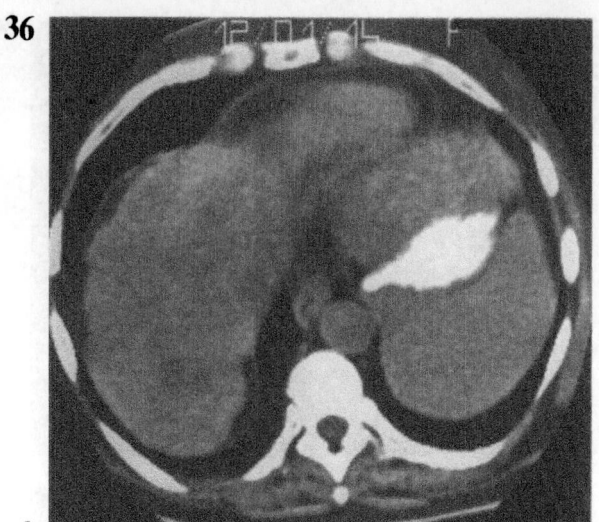

Inj.

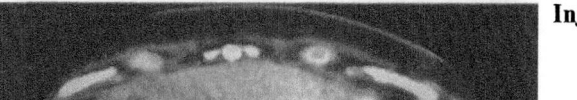

32

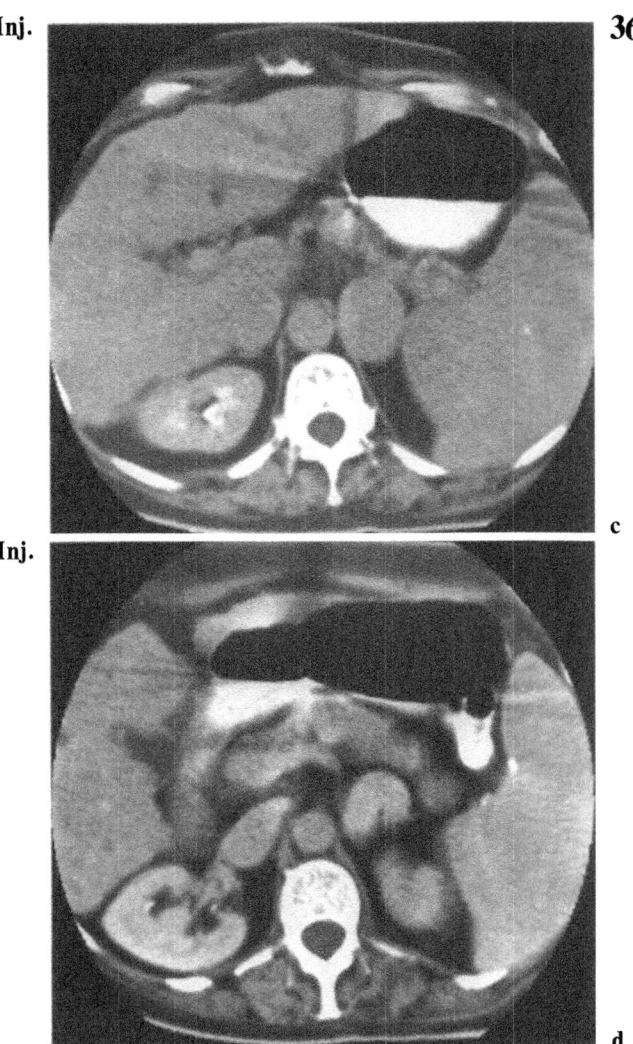

Inj.

36

c

Inj.

d

37

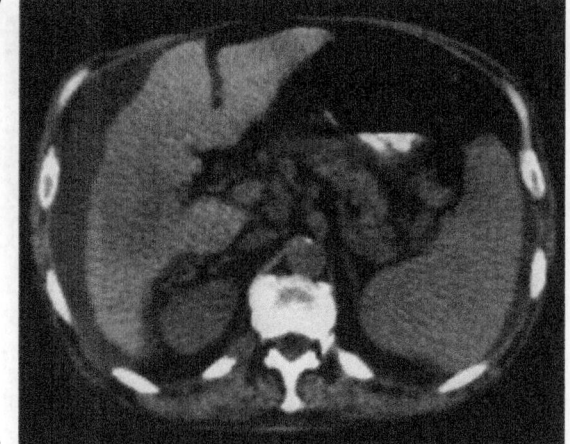

Inj.

a

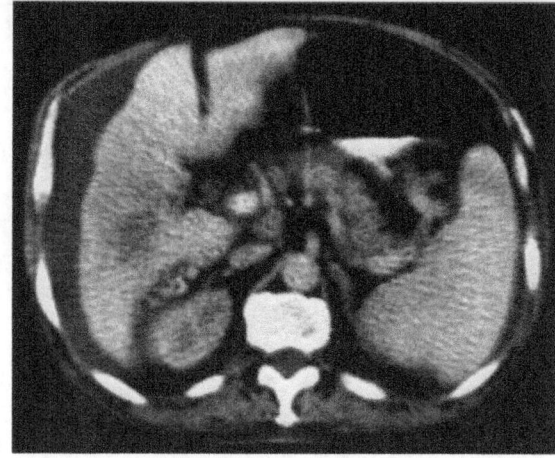

b

38

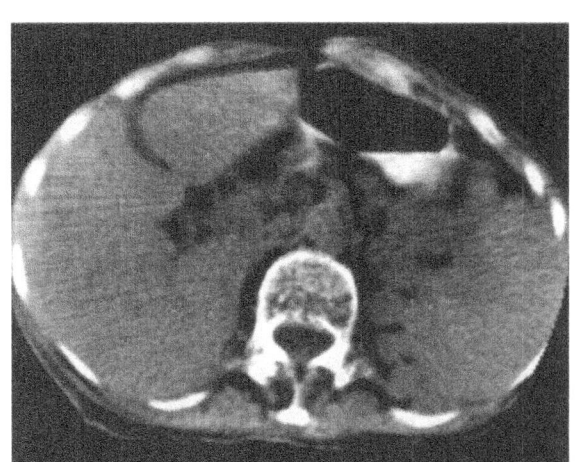

Inj.

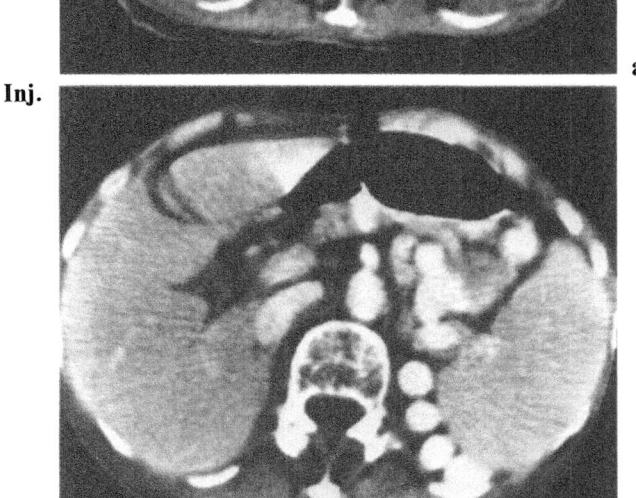

a

b

39

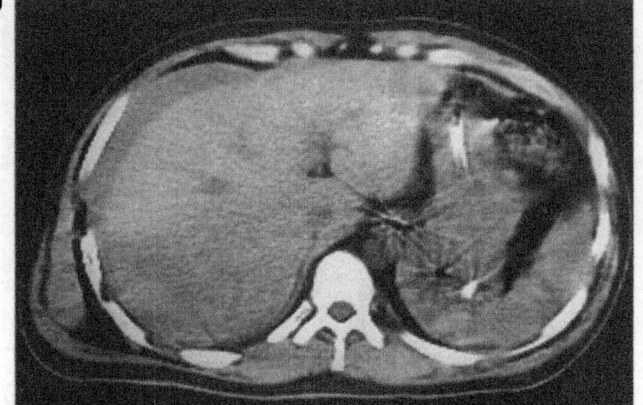

a

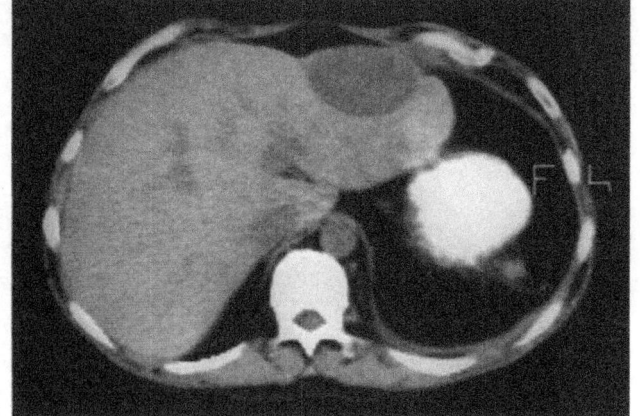

b

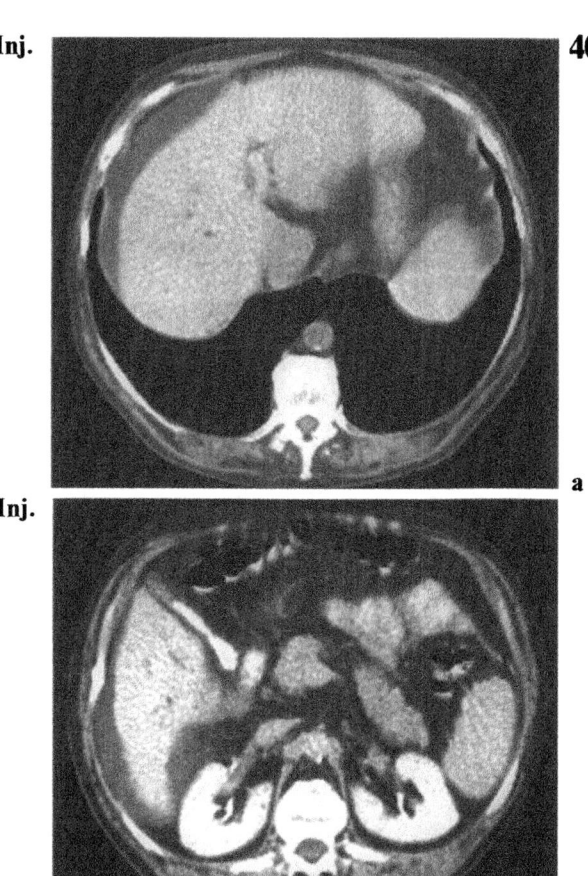

a

b

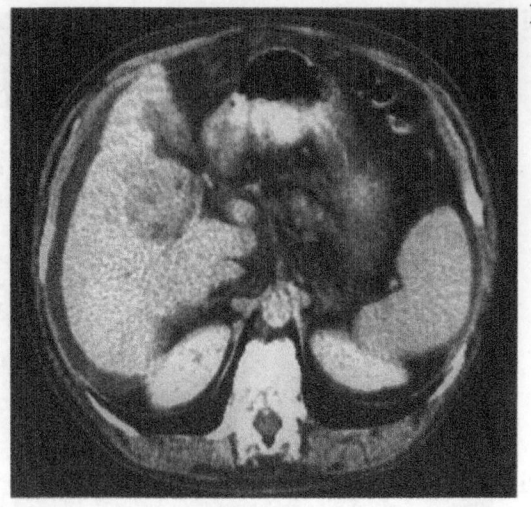

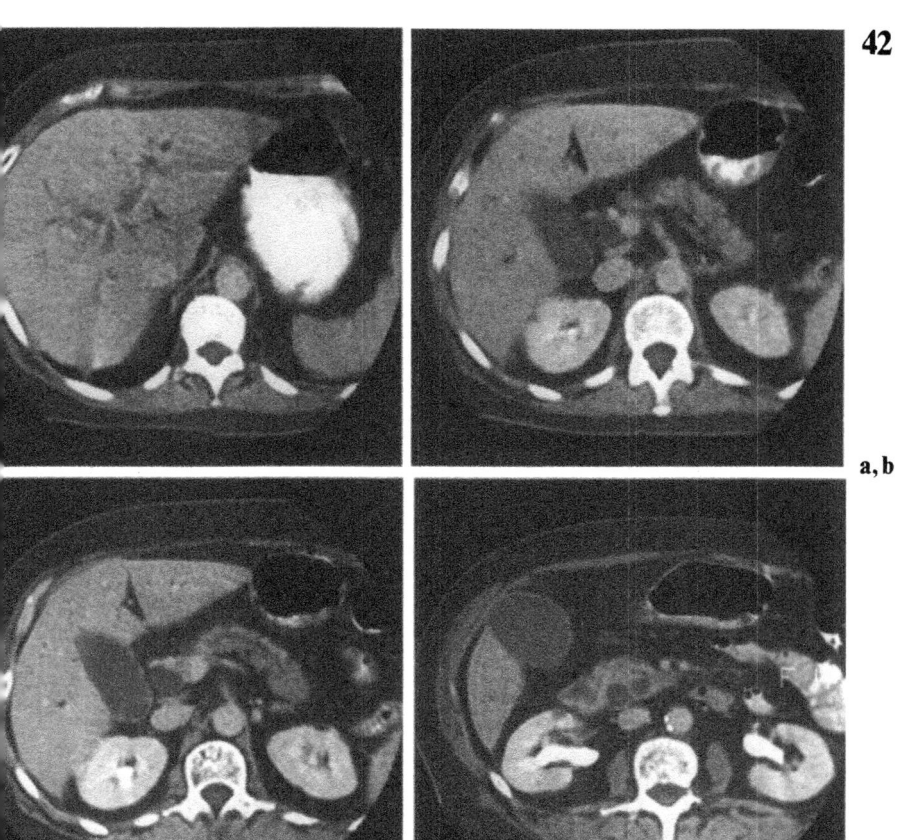

a, b

c, d

Inj.

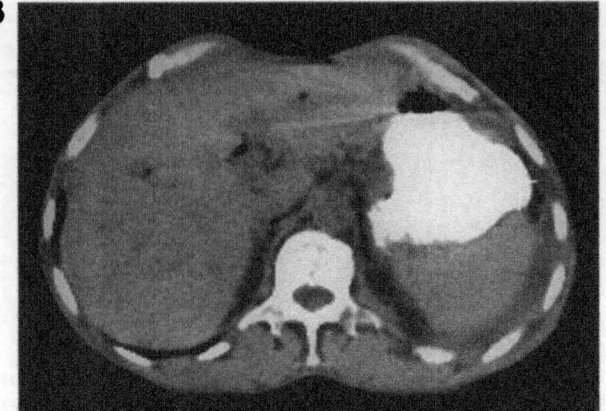

Inj.

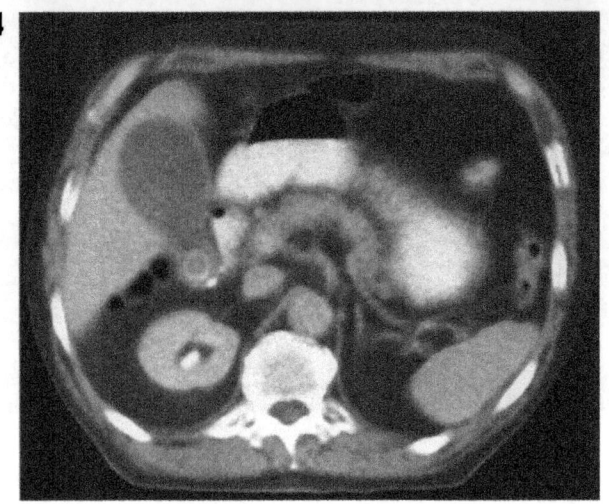

45

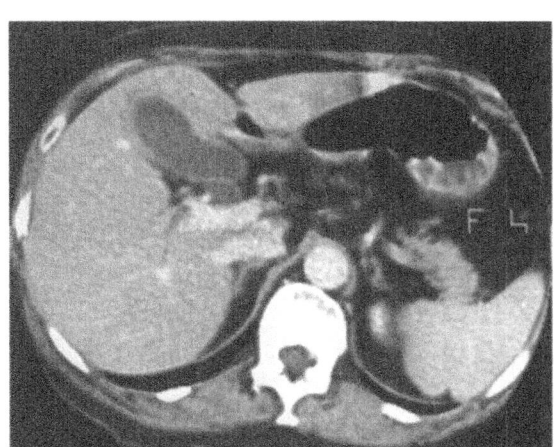

Inj.

a

b

46 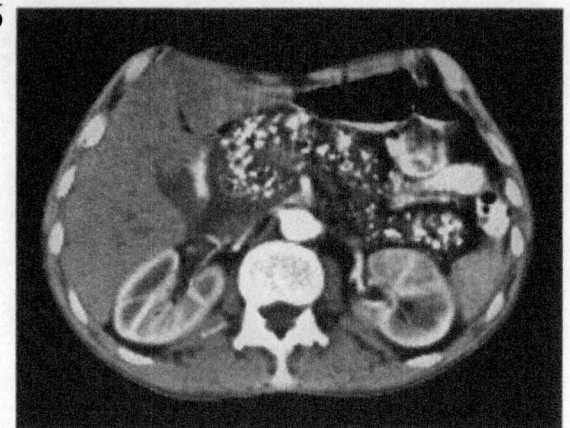 Inj.

47 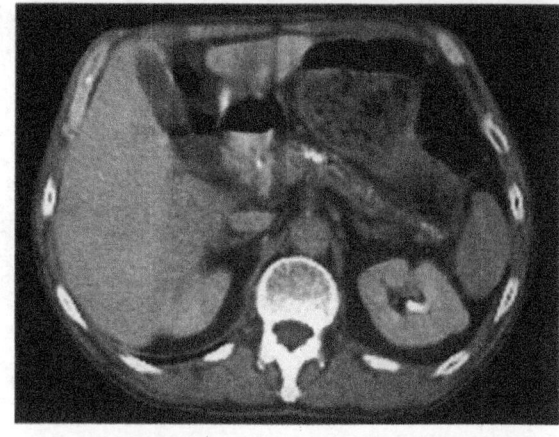 Inj.

48 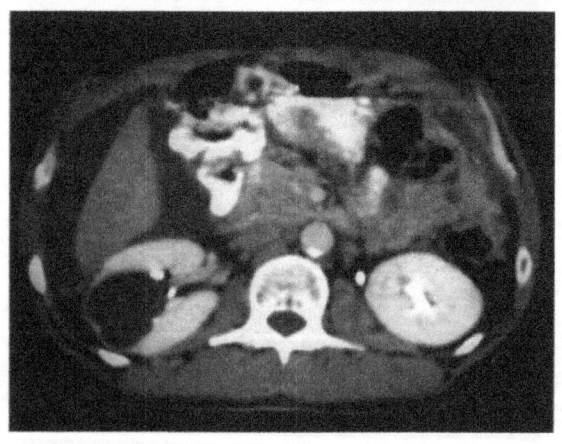 Inj.

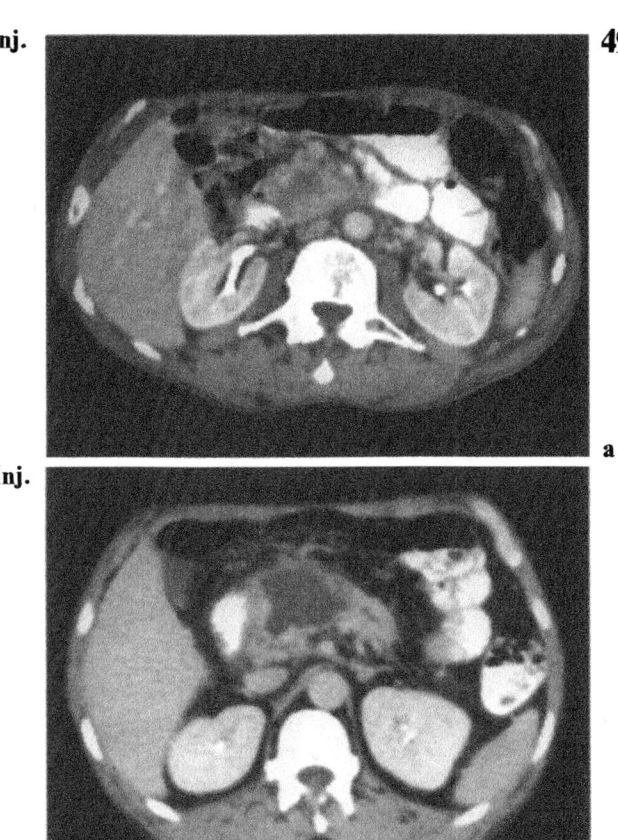

a

b

50

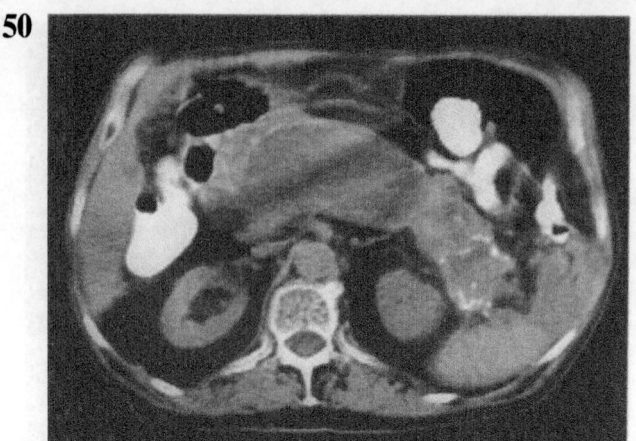

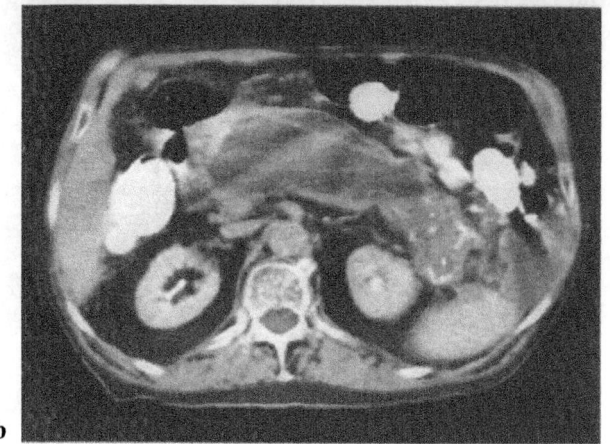

a

b

Inj.

Inj.

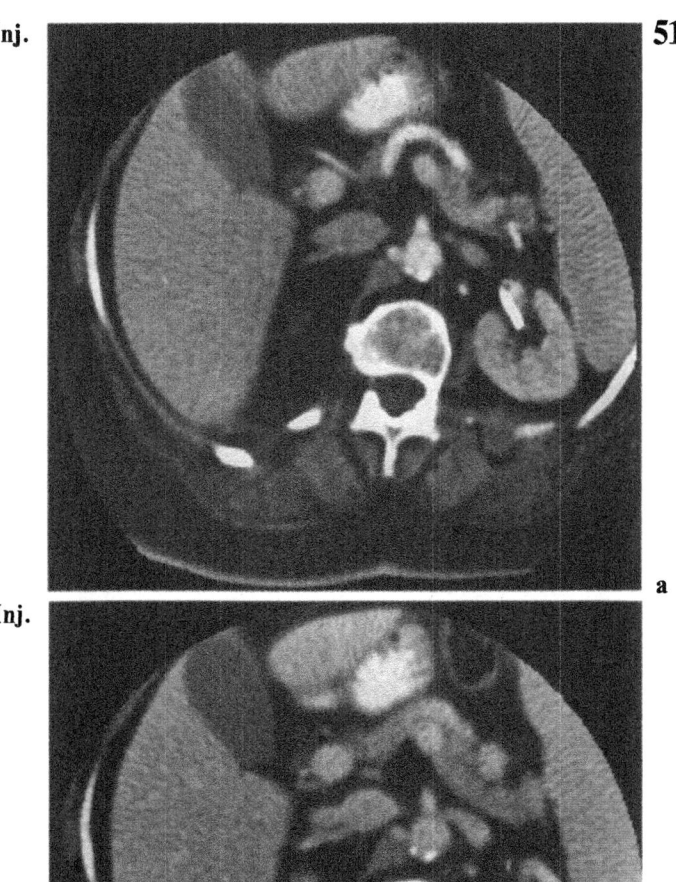

a

Inj.

b

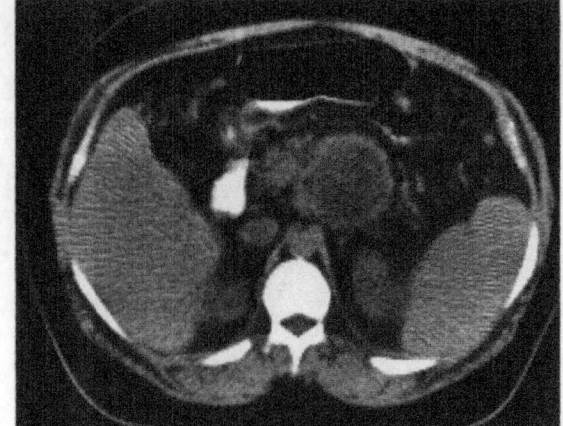

a

Inj.

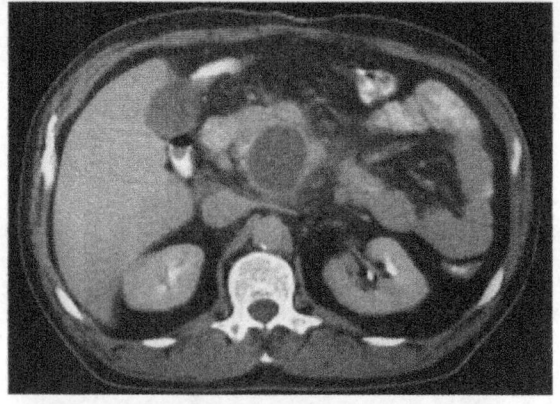

b

Inj.

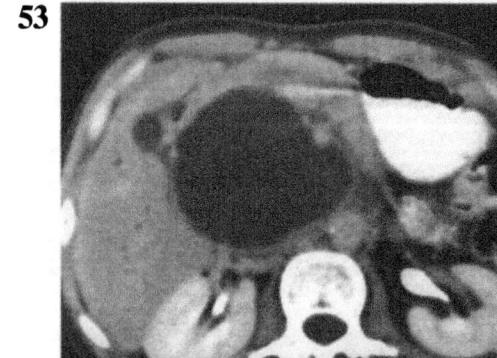

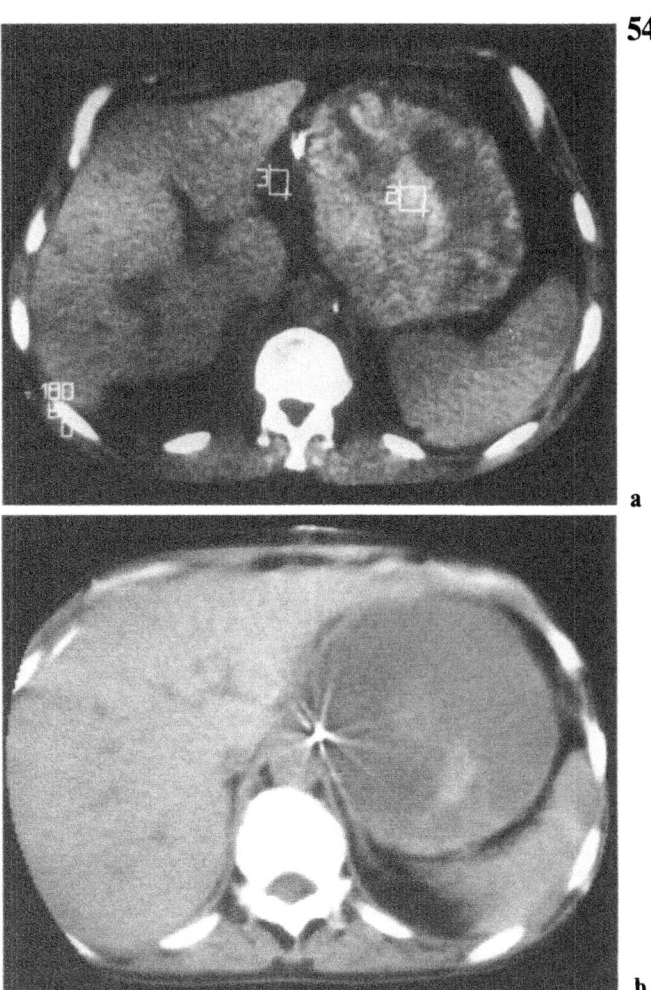

55

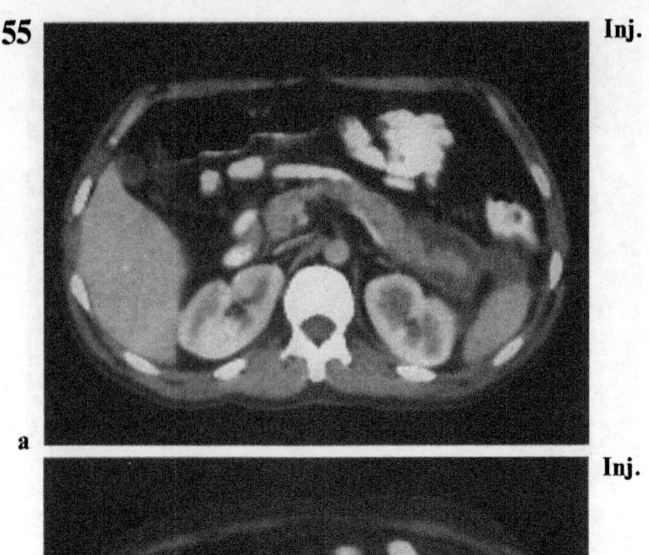

a

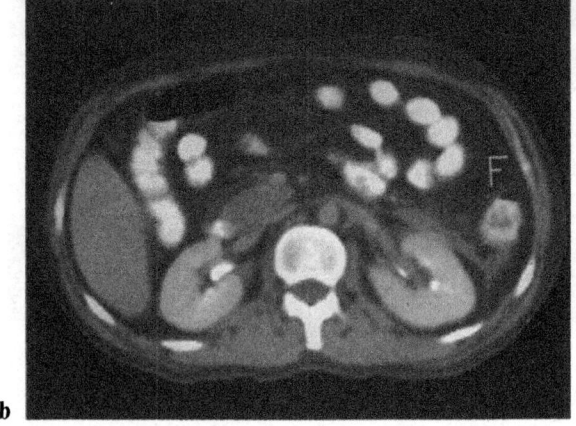

b

Inj.

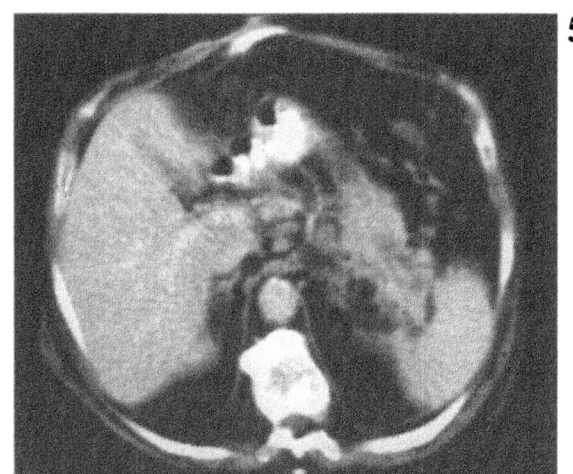

Inj.

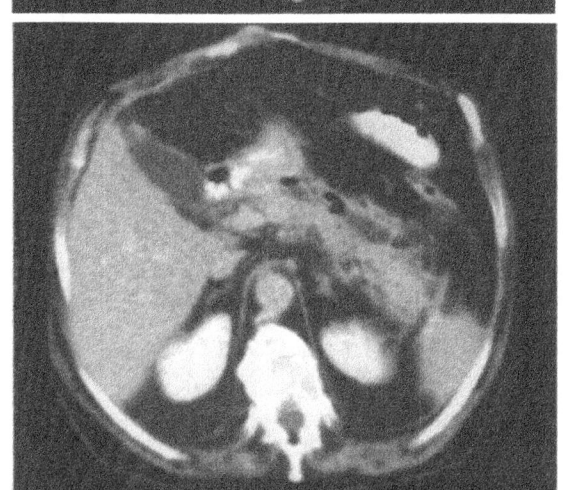

Inj.

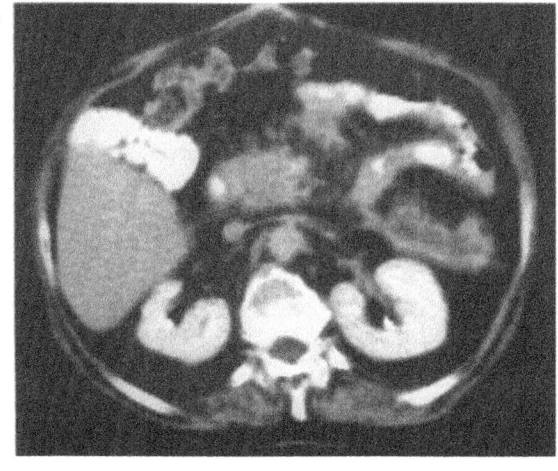

56

Inj.

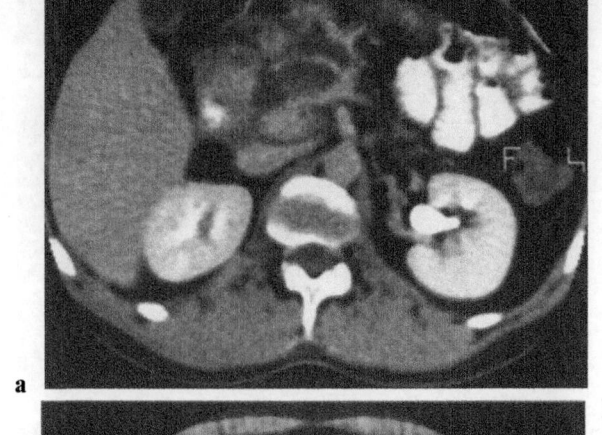

a

Inj.

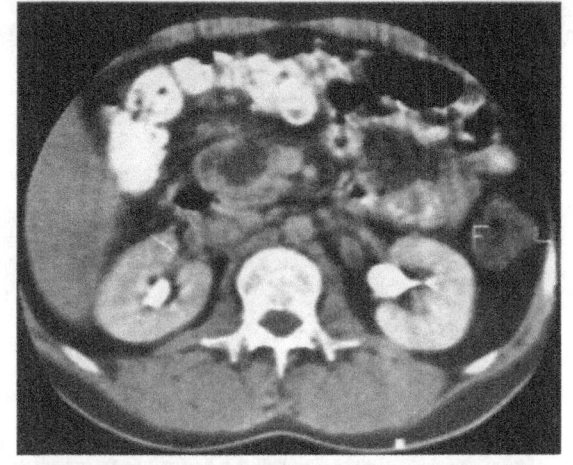

b

Inj.

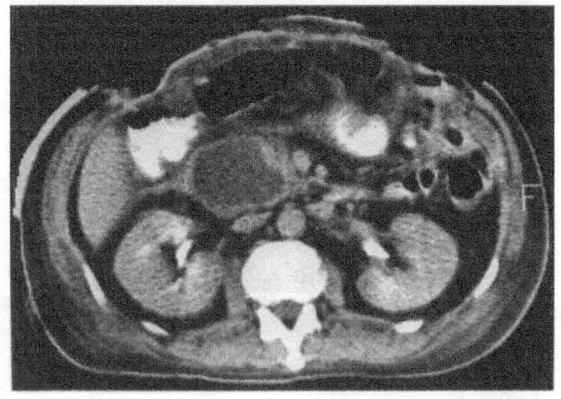

c

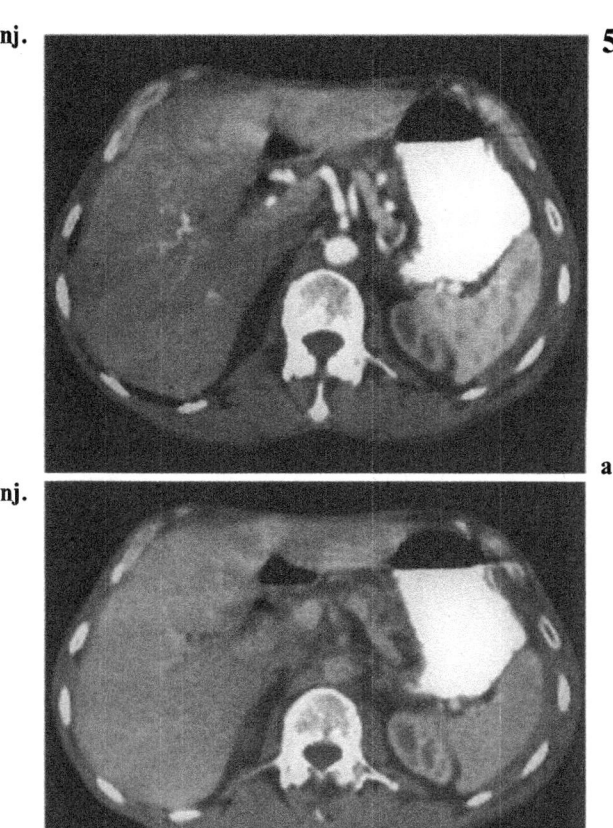

a

b

58

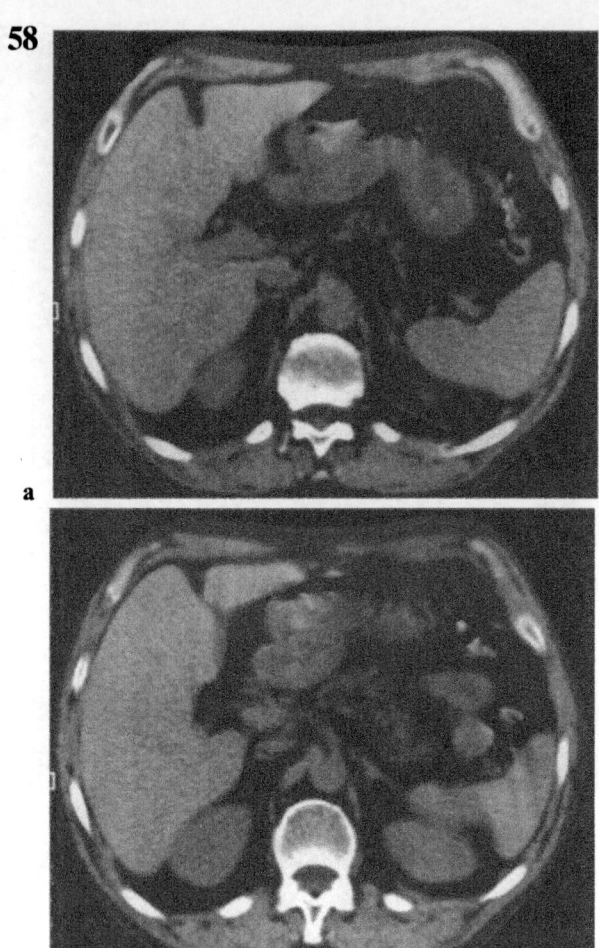

a

b

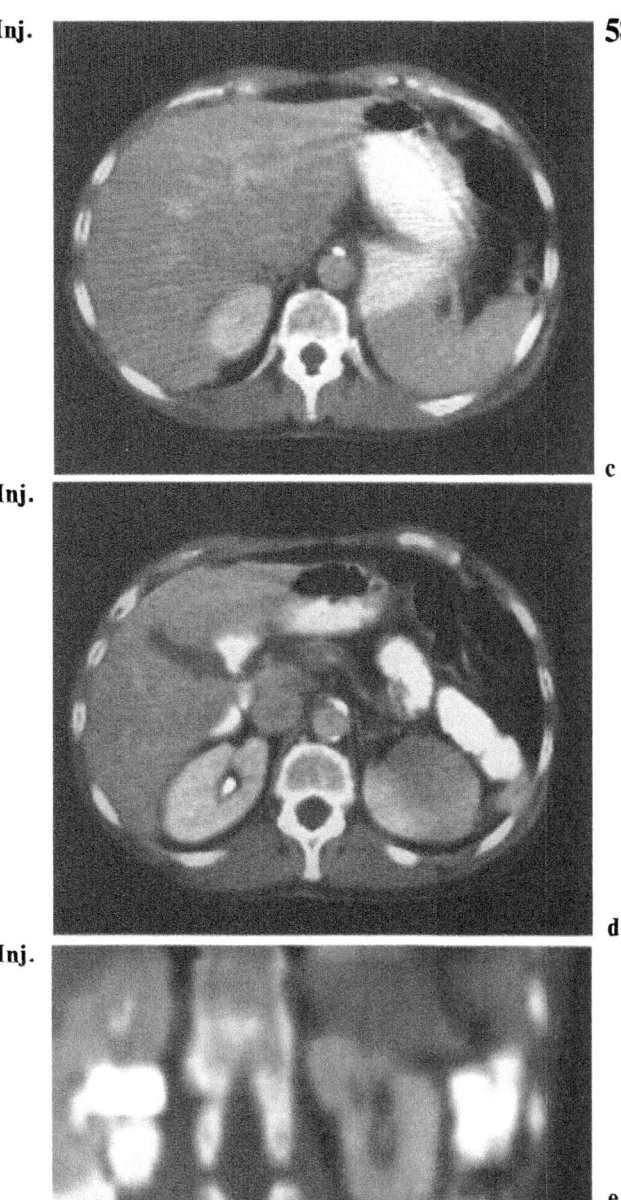

Inj.

58

Inj.

c

Inj.

d

e

59

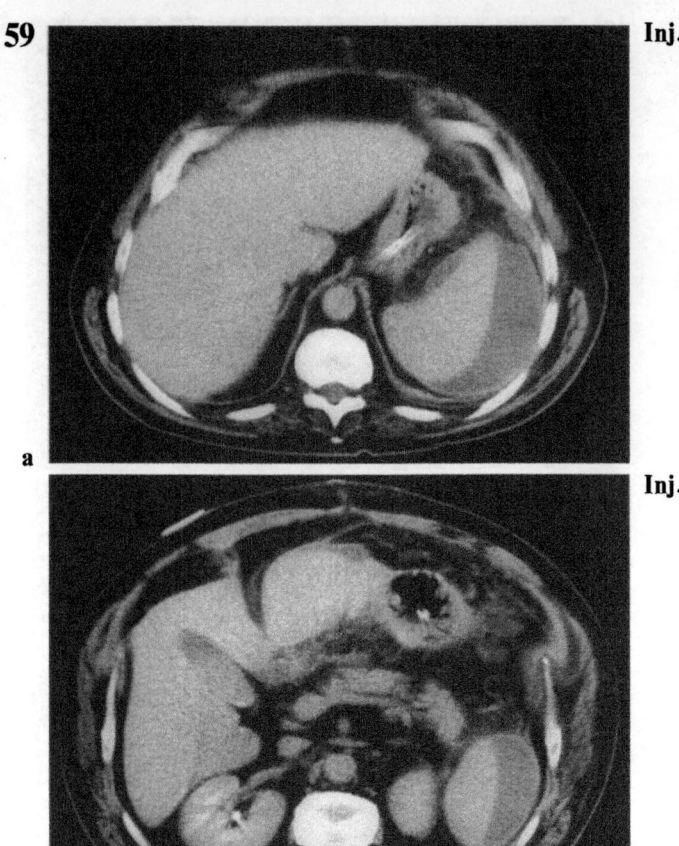

a

b

Inj.

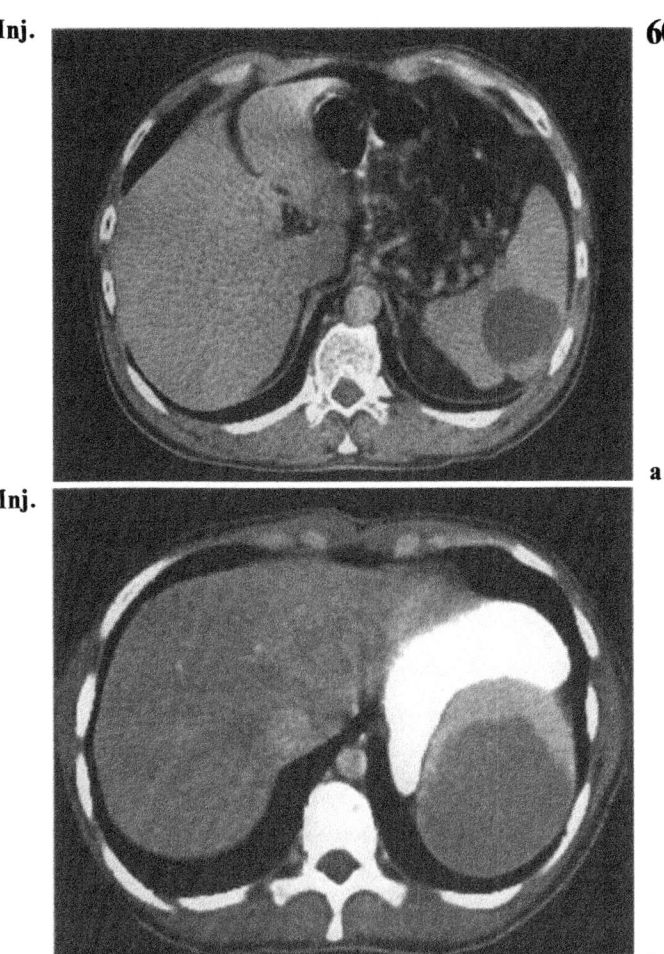

Inj.

a

b

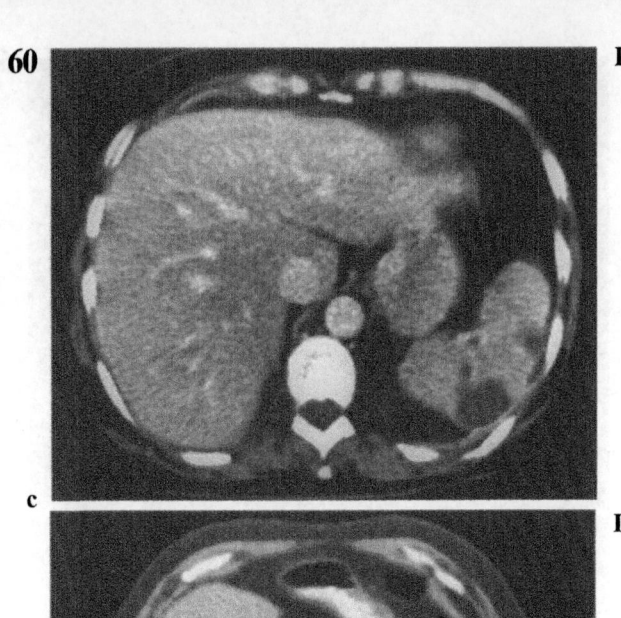

Inj.

c

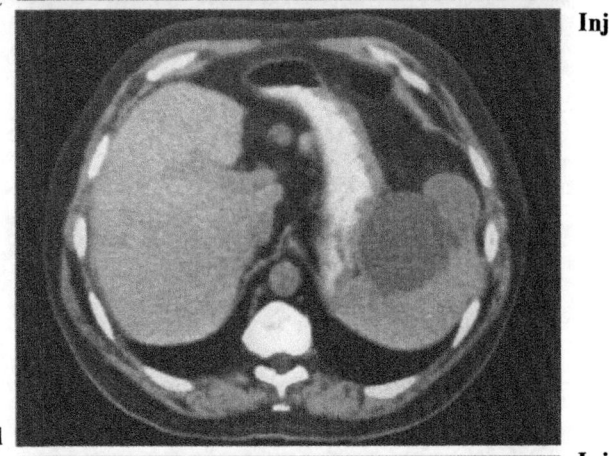

Inj.

d

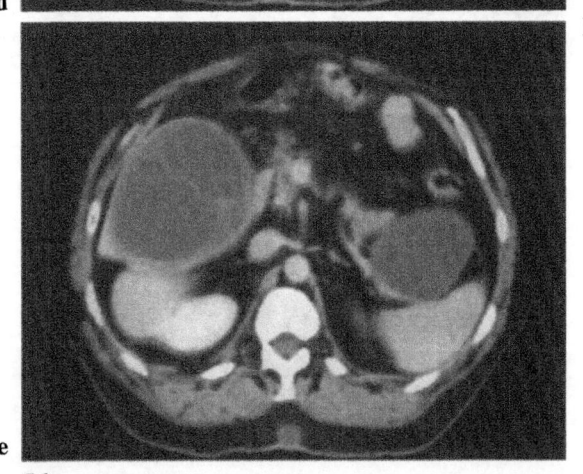

Inj.

e

Inj.   **61**

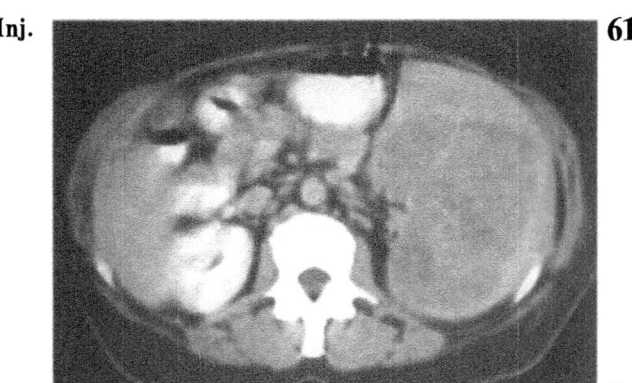

a

Inj.

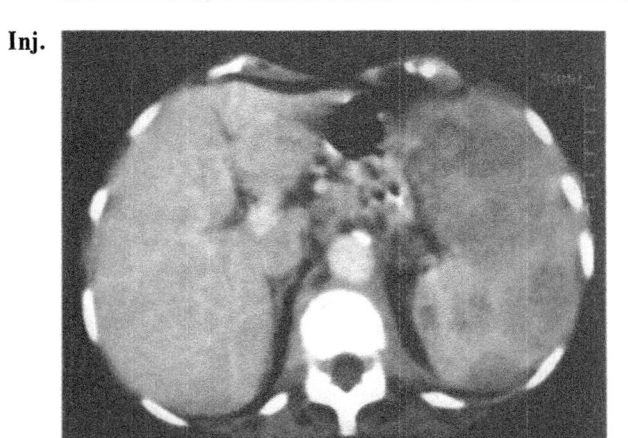

b

62

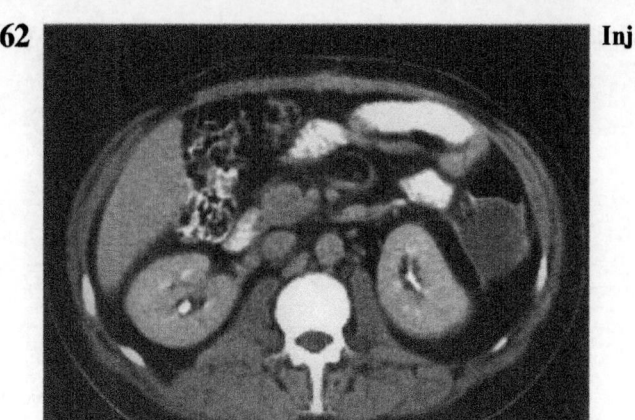

a

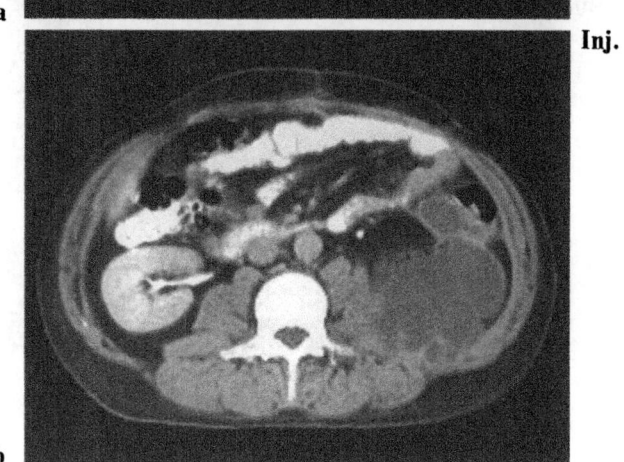

b

Inj.

Inj.

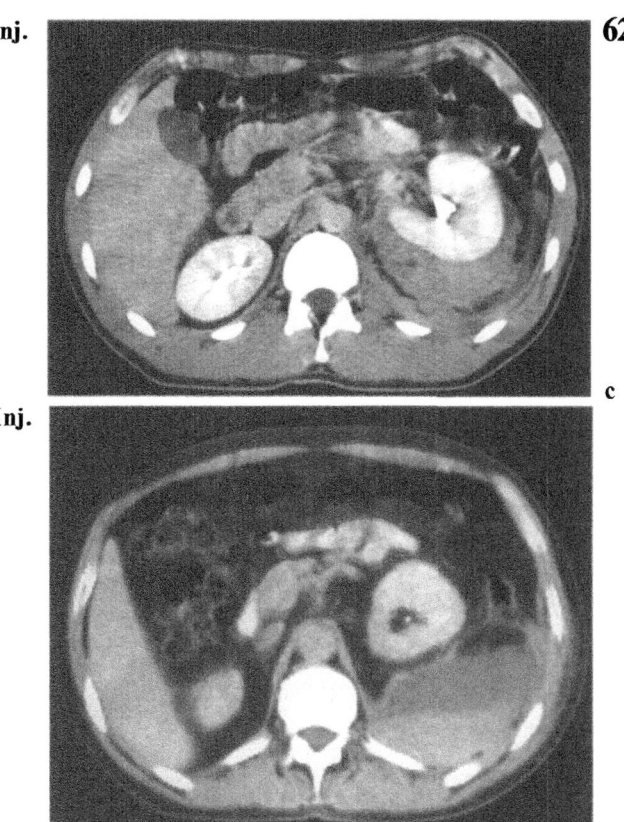

c

d

63

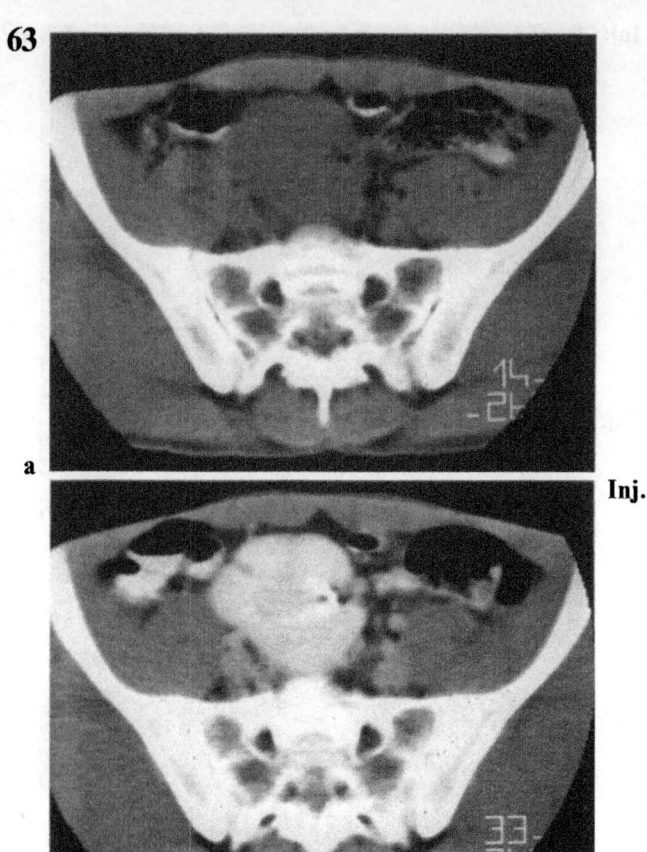

a

Inj.

b

Inj.

63

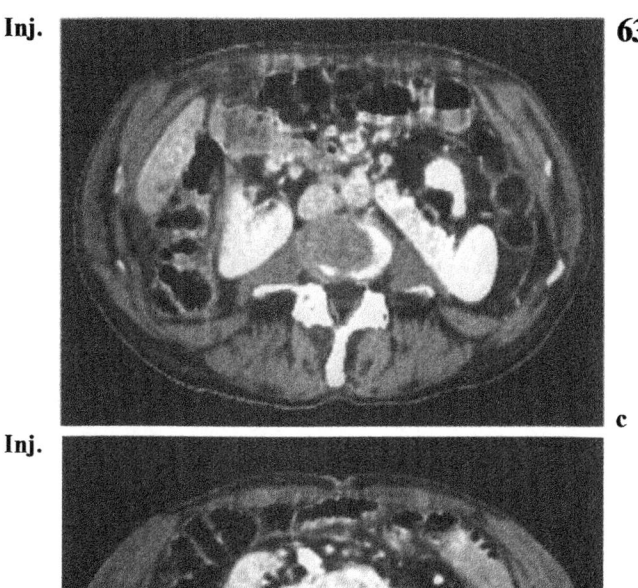

c

Inj.

d

63

Inj.

Inj.

Inj.

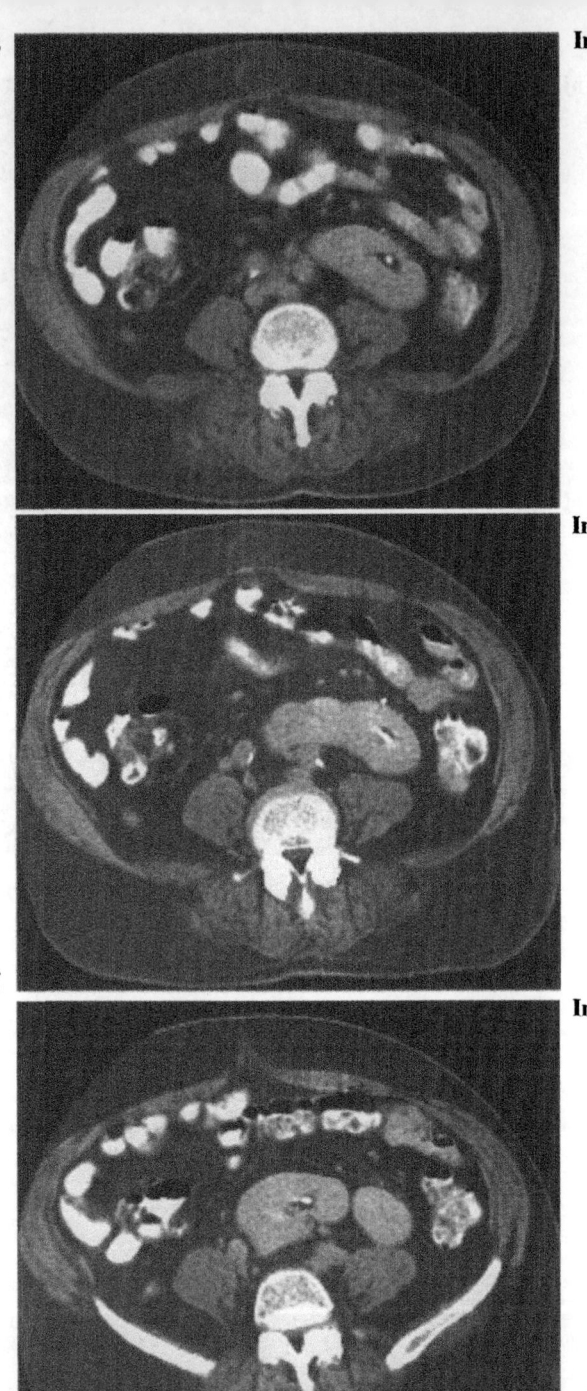

e

f

g

Inj.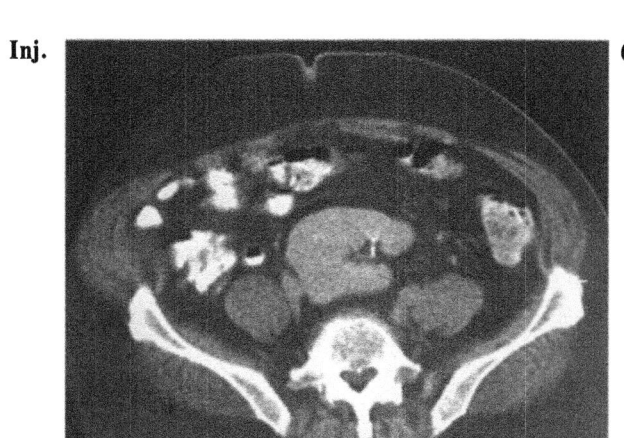

h

Inj.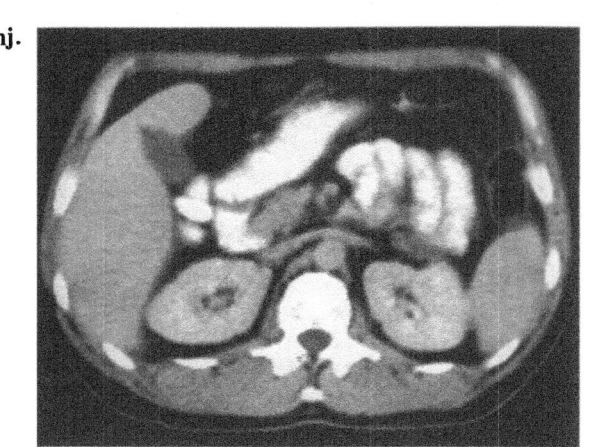

i

64   Inj.

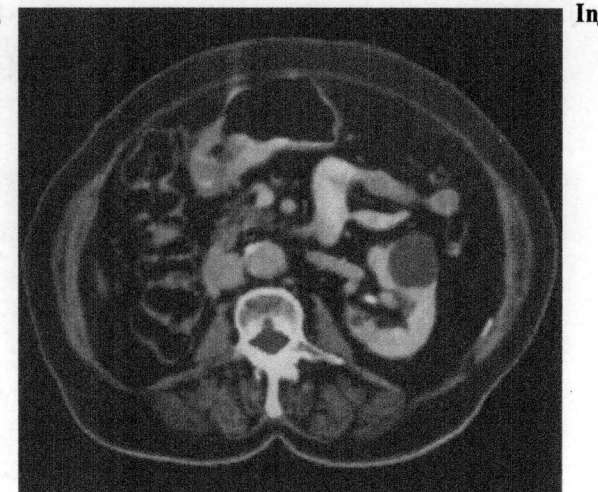

65   Inj.

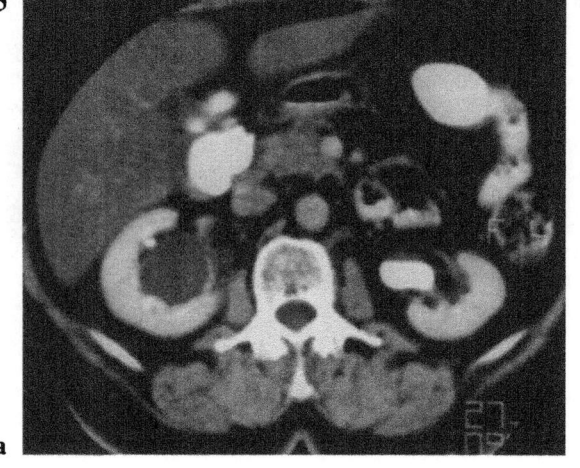

a

Inj.

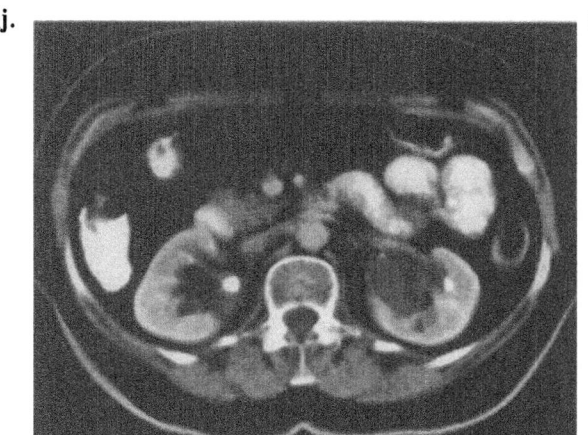

b

Inj.

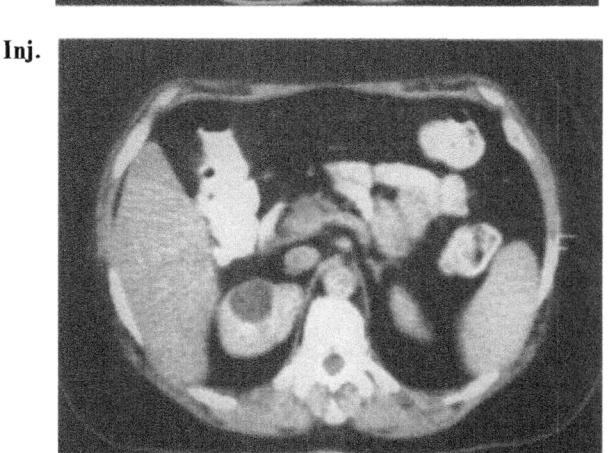

c

Inj.

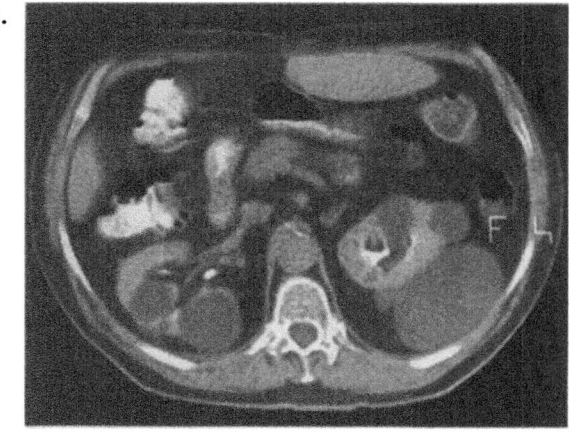

d

66

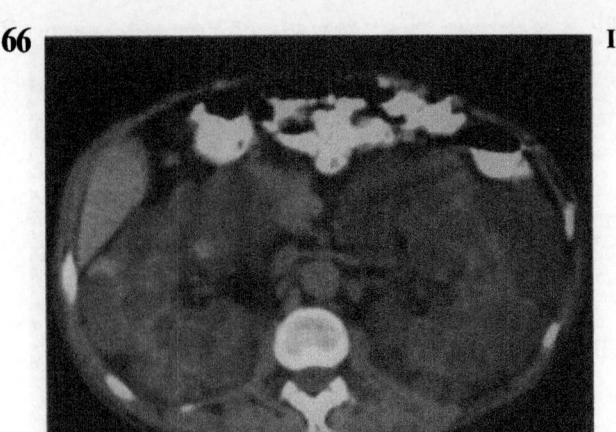

a

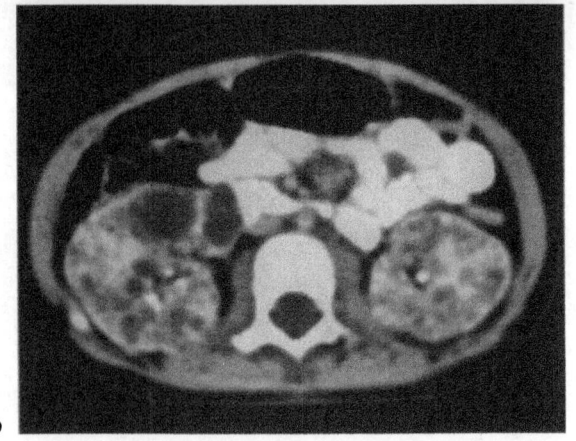

b

67

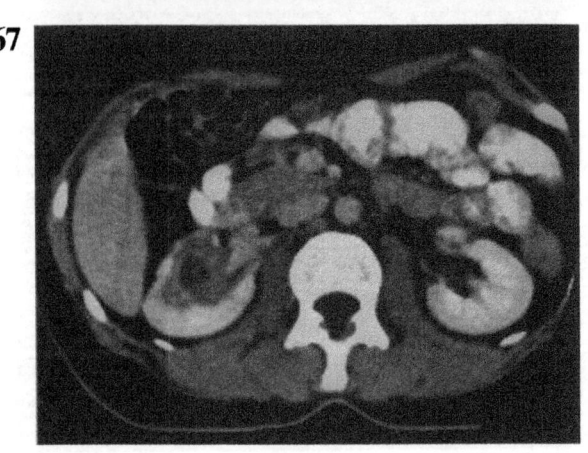

68

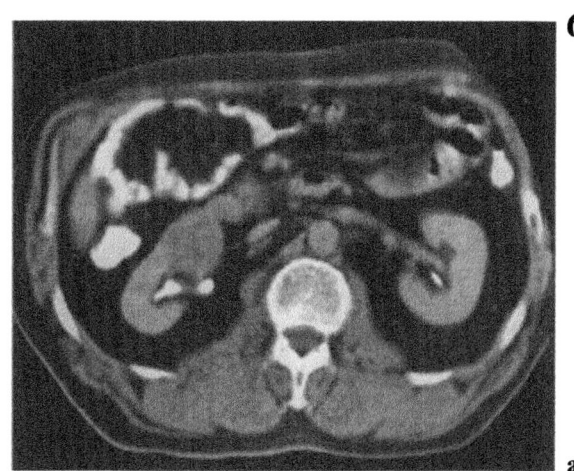

Inj.

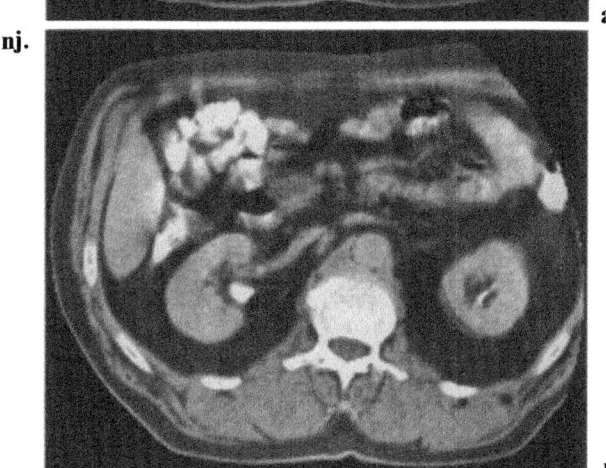

a

b

68

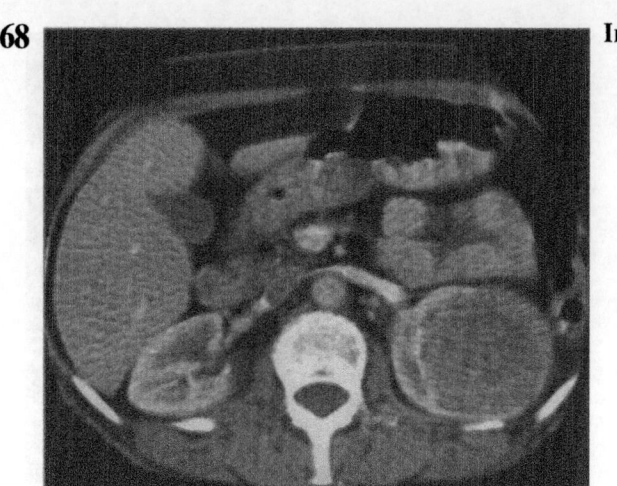

c

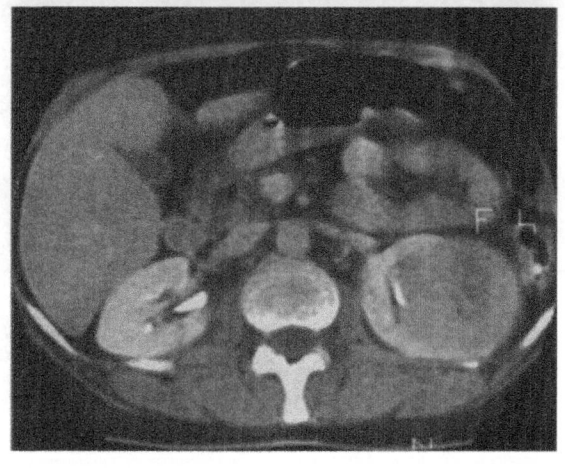

d

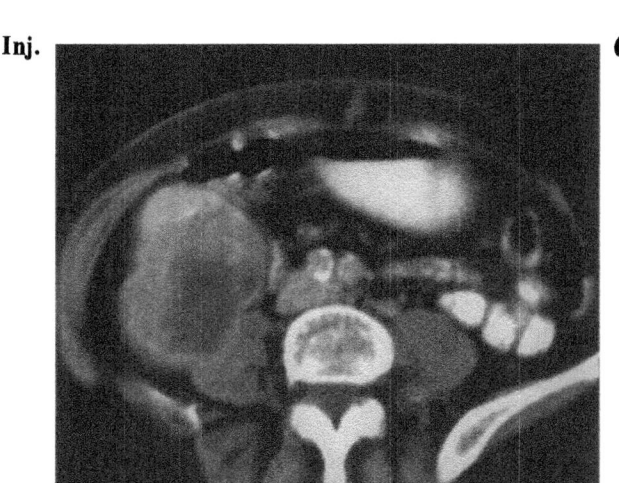

a

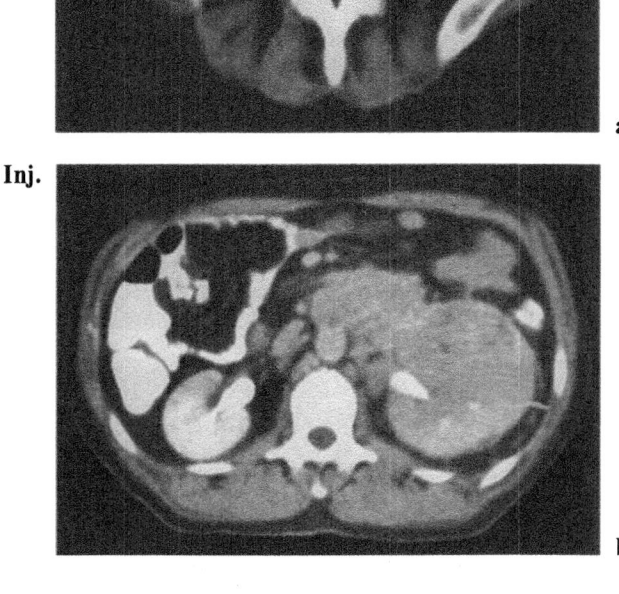

b

70

In

Inj.

In

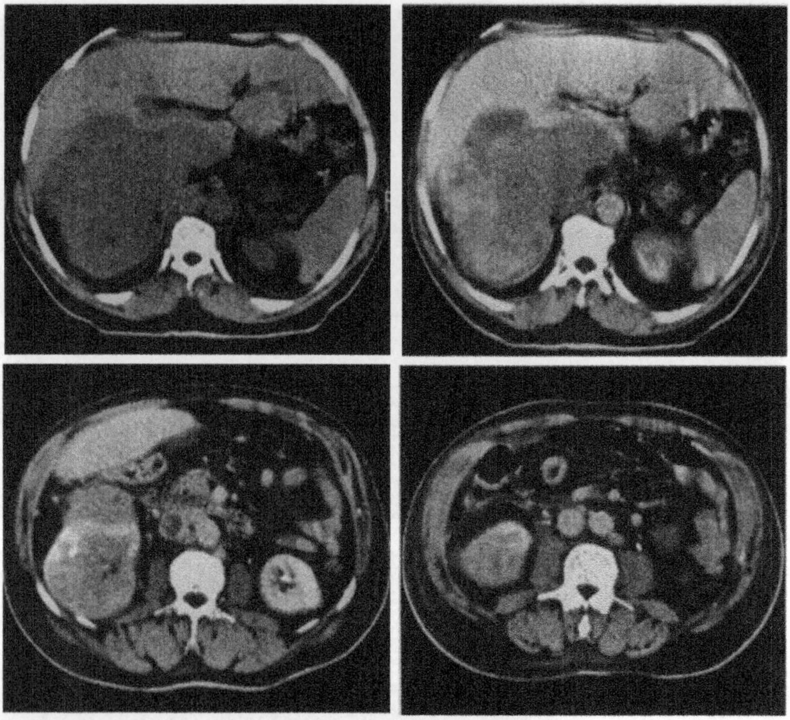

a

Inj.

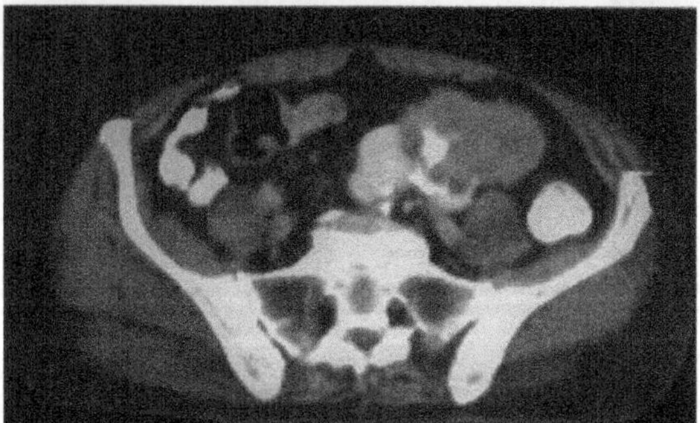

d

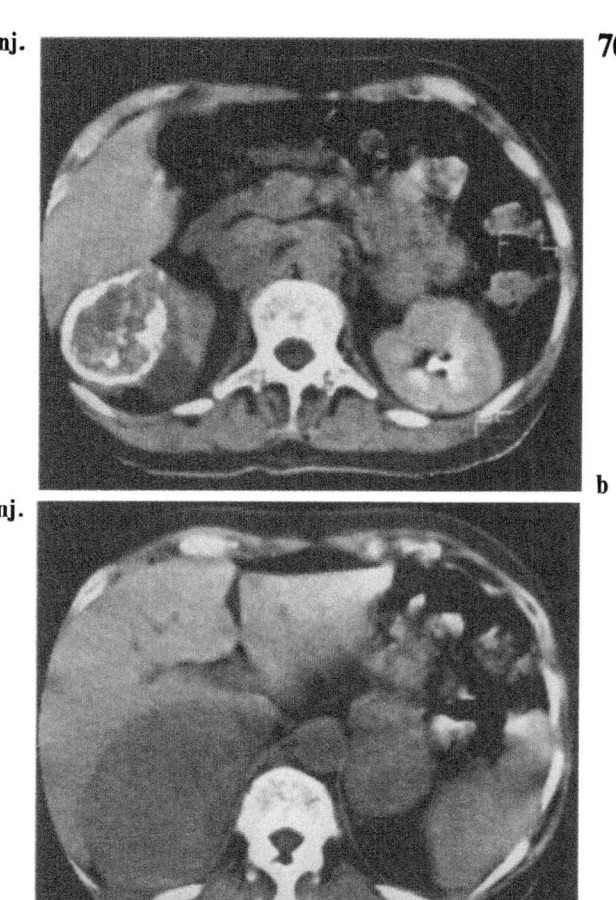

71

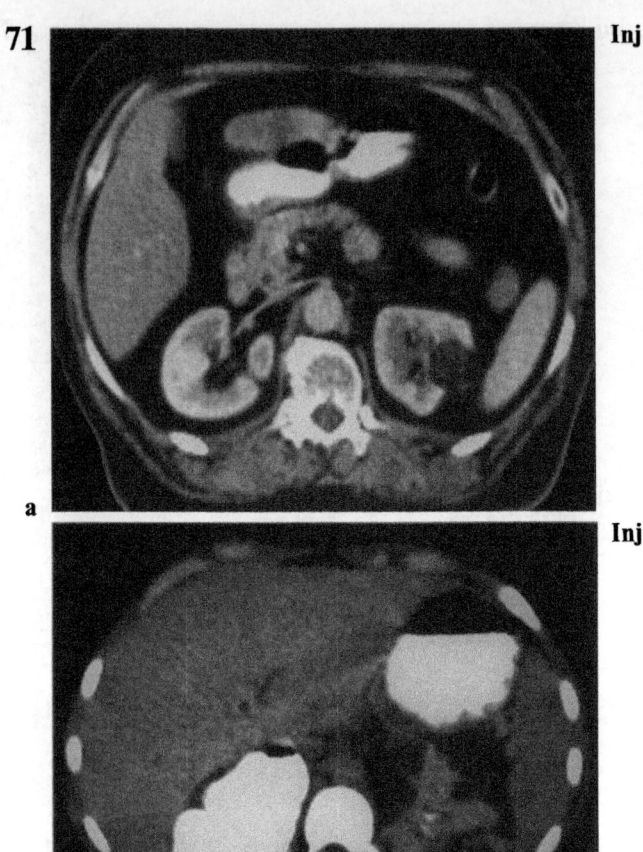

Inj.

Inj.

a

b

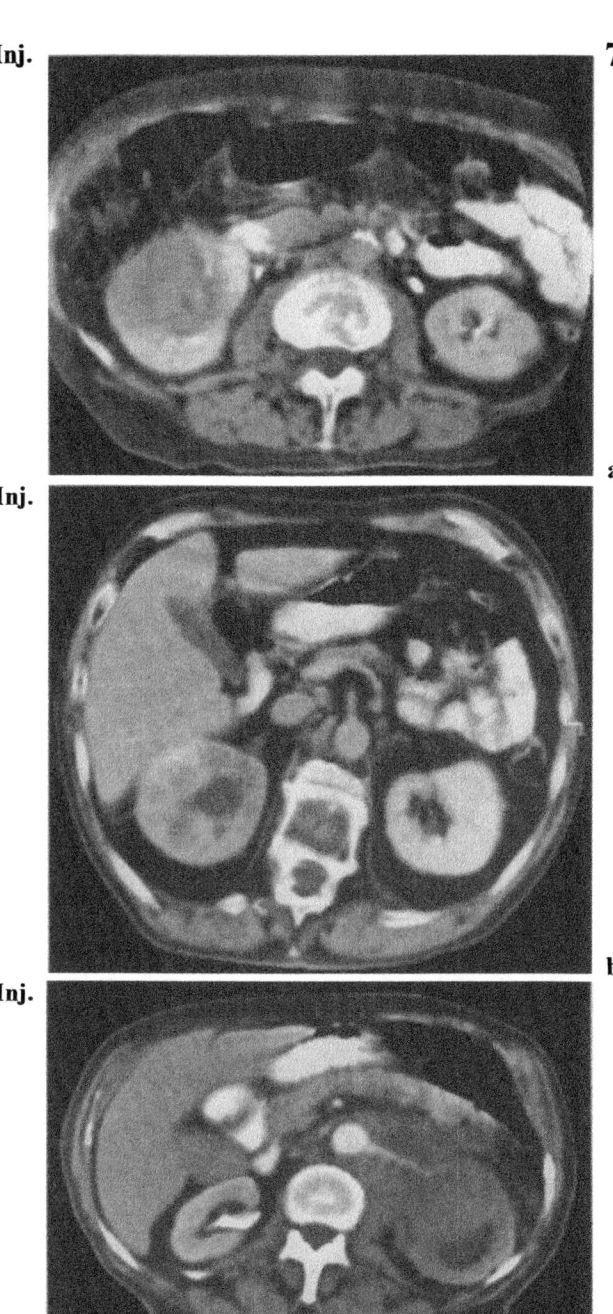

Inj.

a

Inj.

b

Inj.

c

73

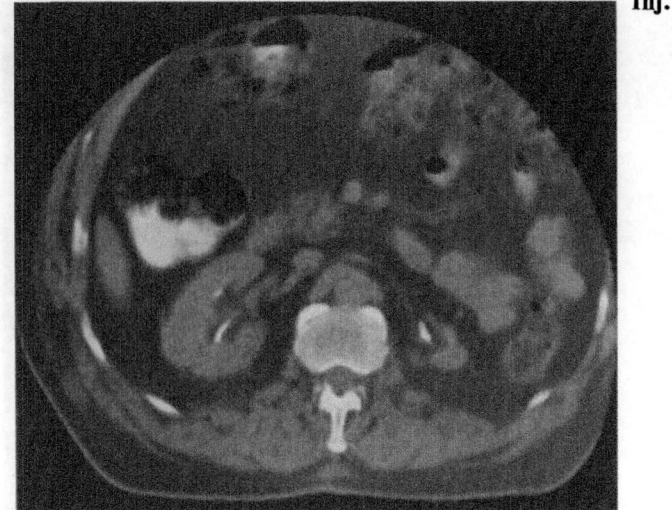

a

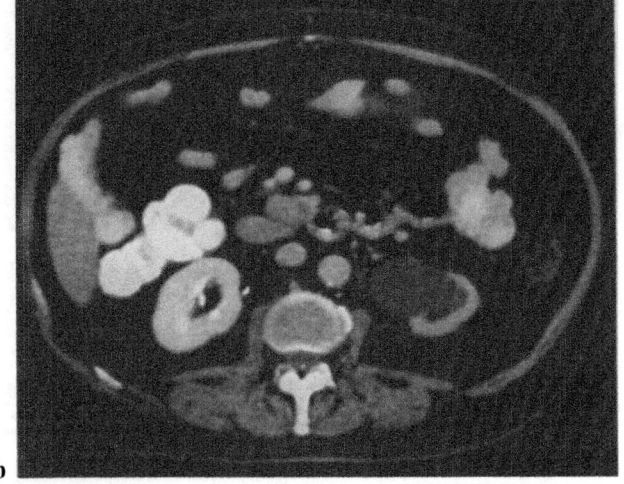

b

74

Inj.

73

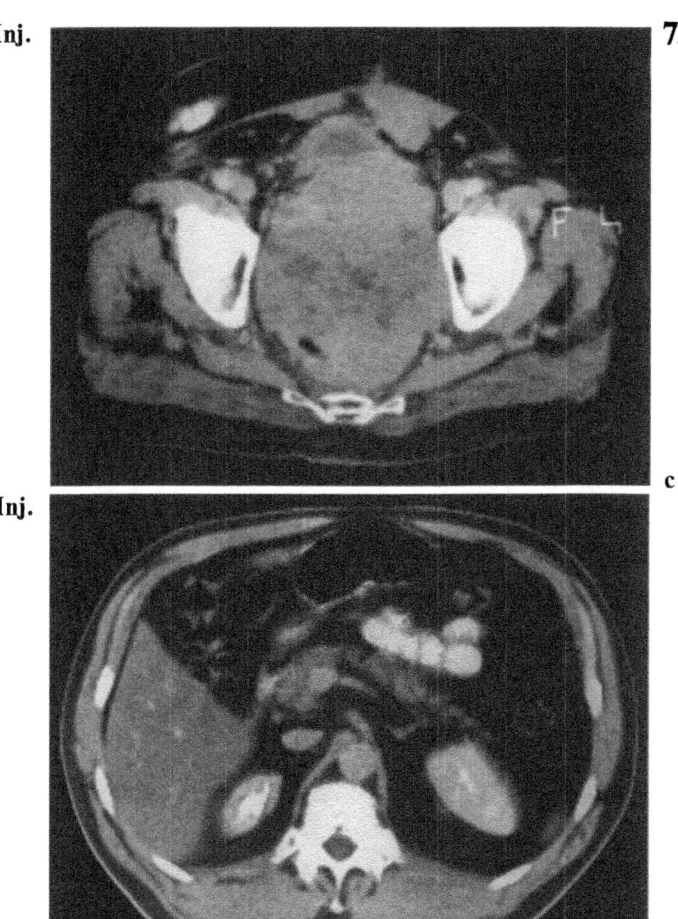

c

Inj.

d

Inj.

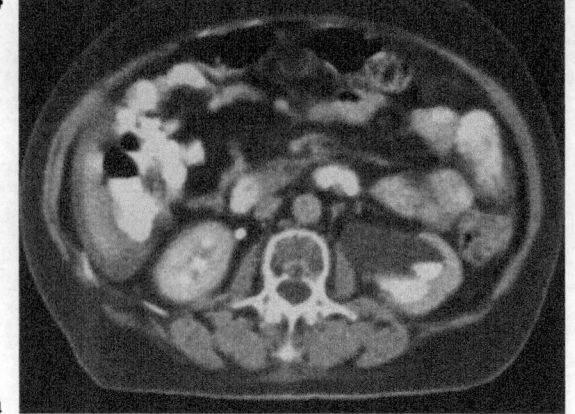

a

Inj.

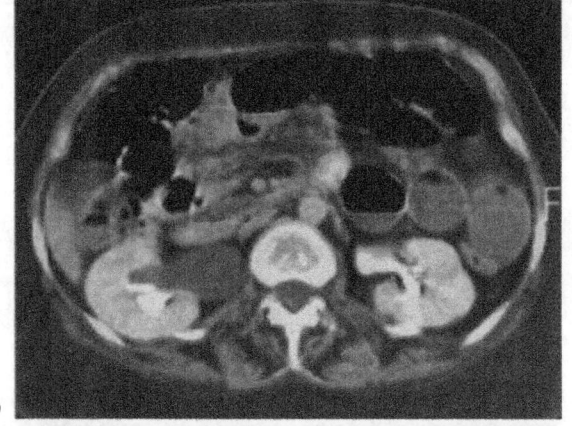

b

Inj.

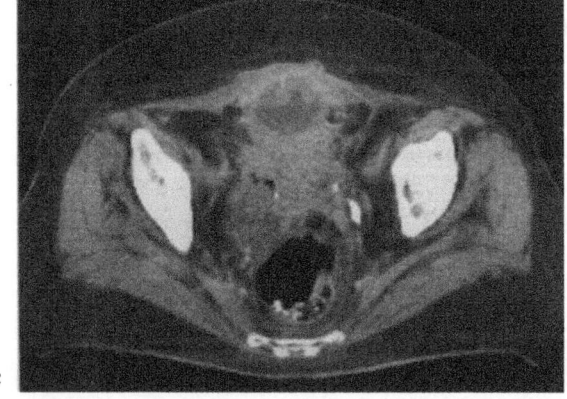

c

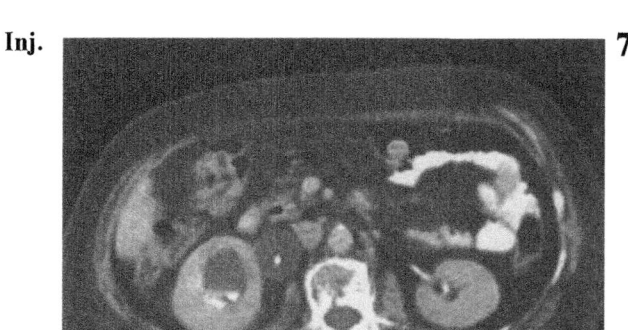

Inj.

74

d

Inj.

e

75

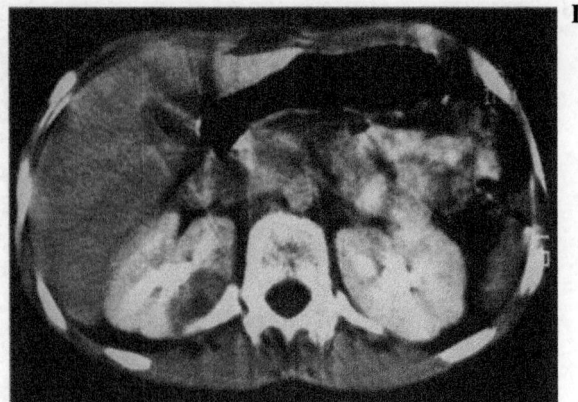

Inj.

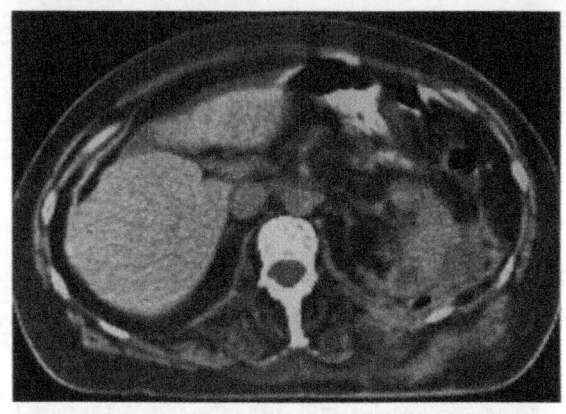

Inj.

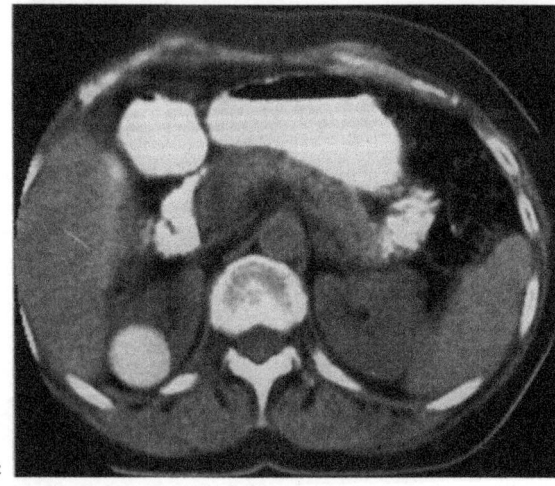

76

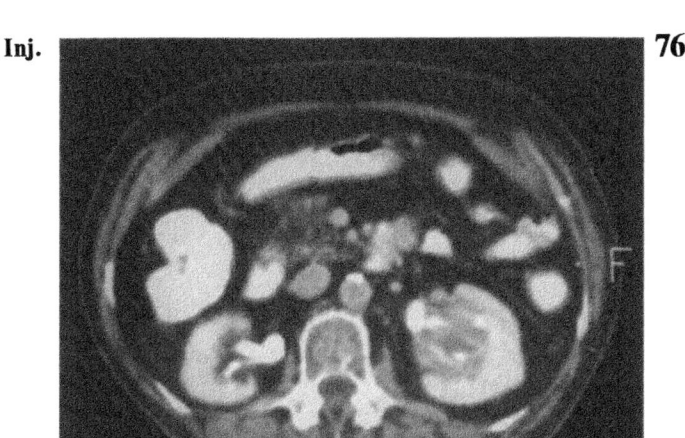

77

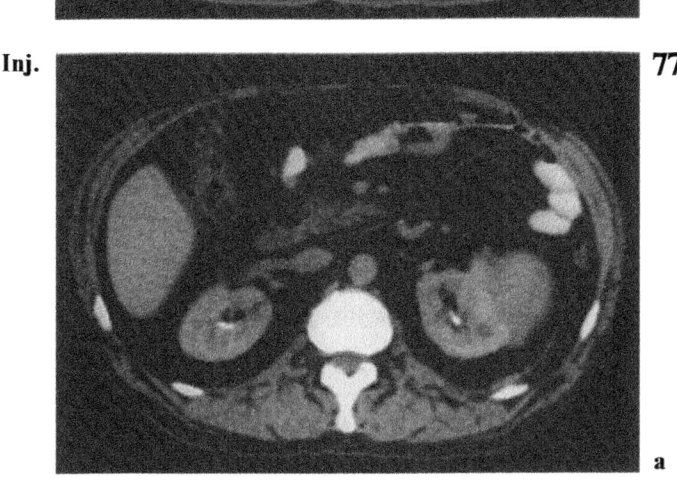

a

79

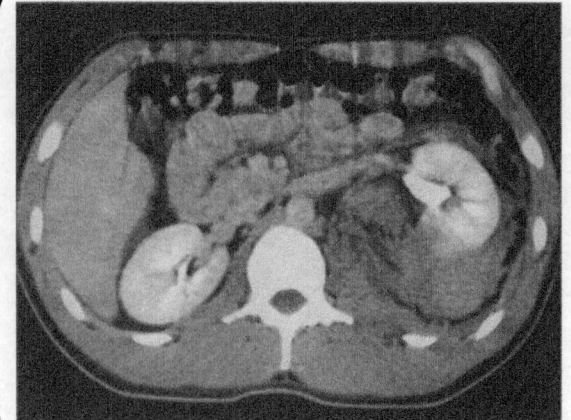
Inj.

b

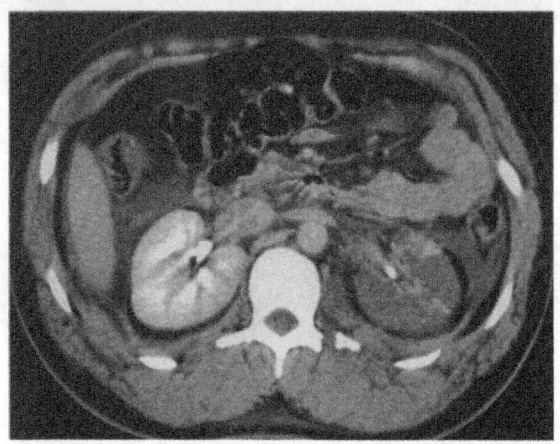
Inj.

c

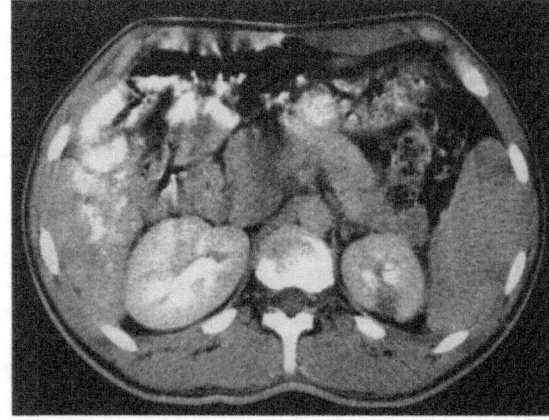
Inj.

d

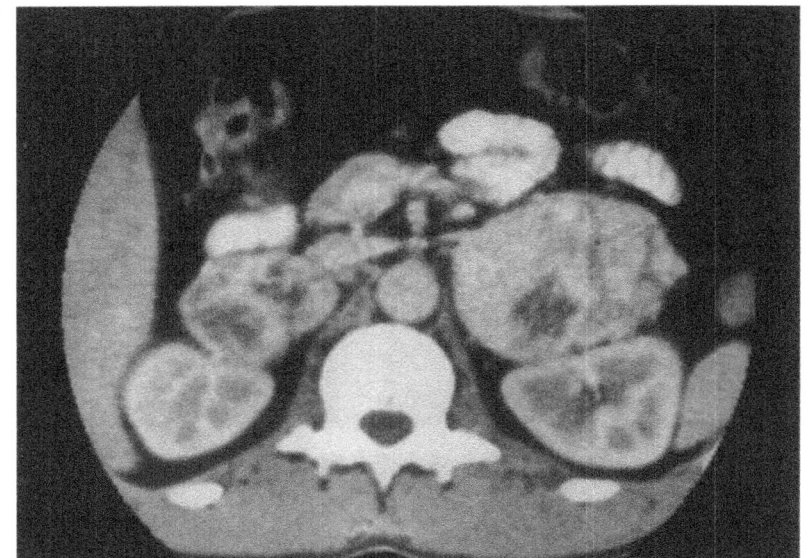

a

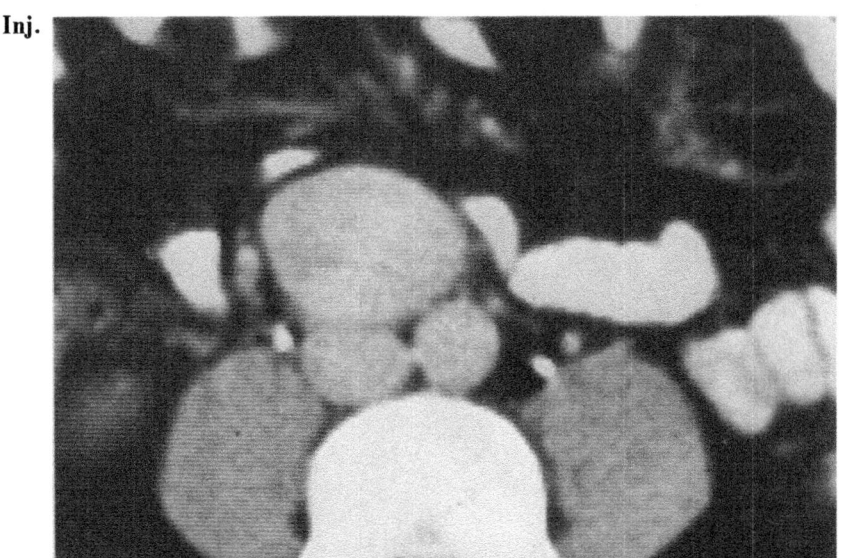

b

79

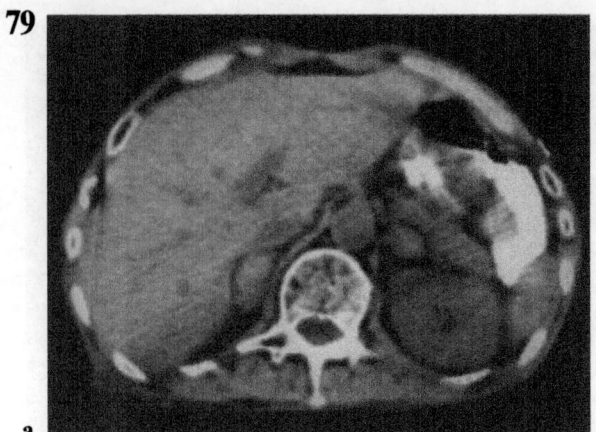

Inj.

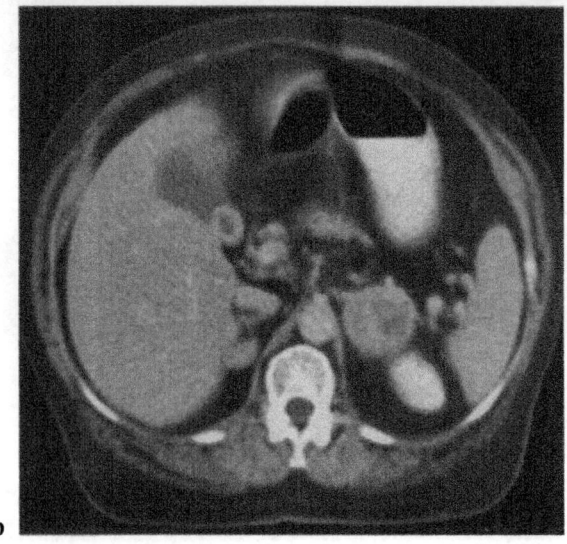

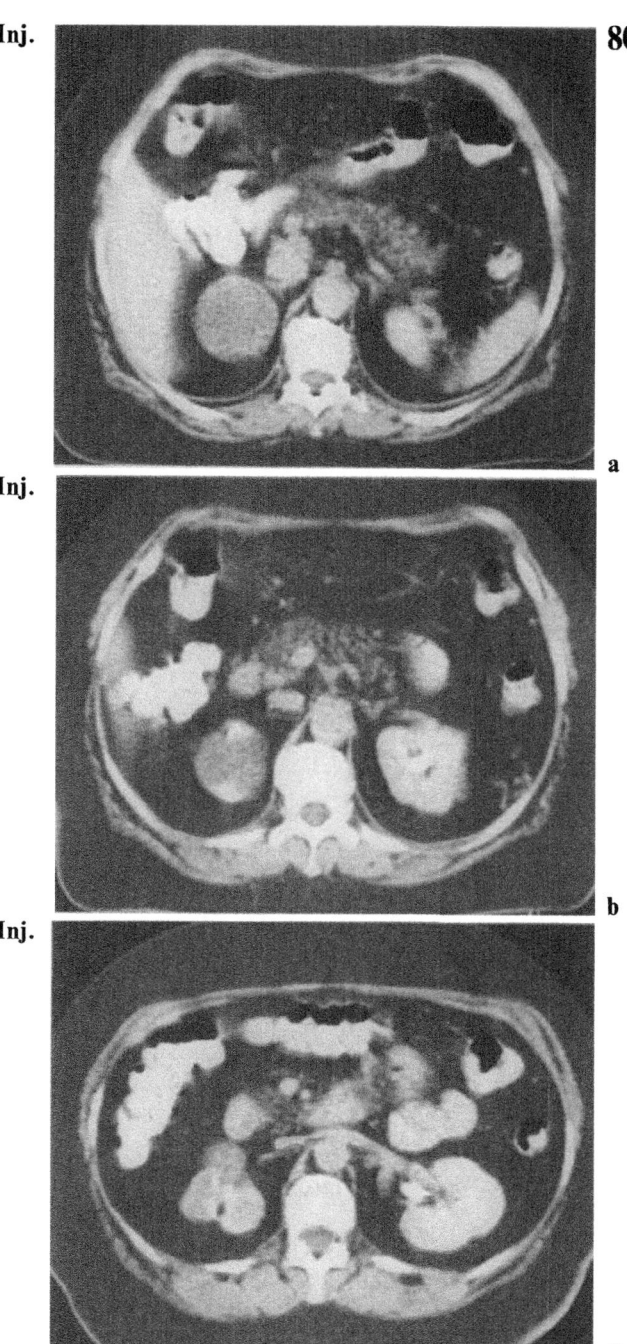

Inj.

a

Inj.

b

Inj.

c

Inj.

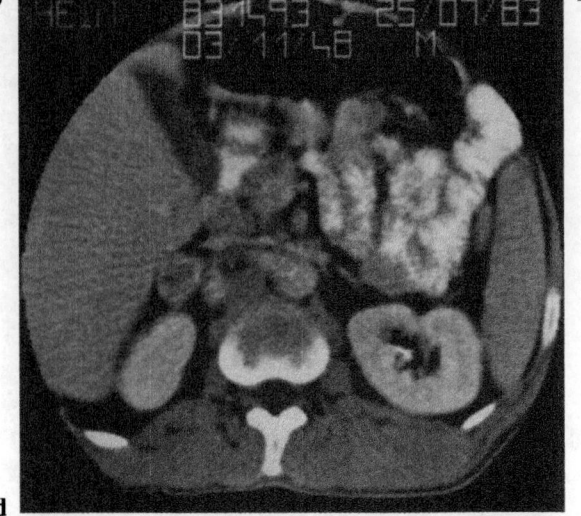

d

Inj.

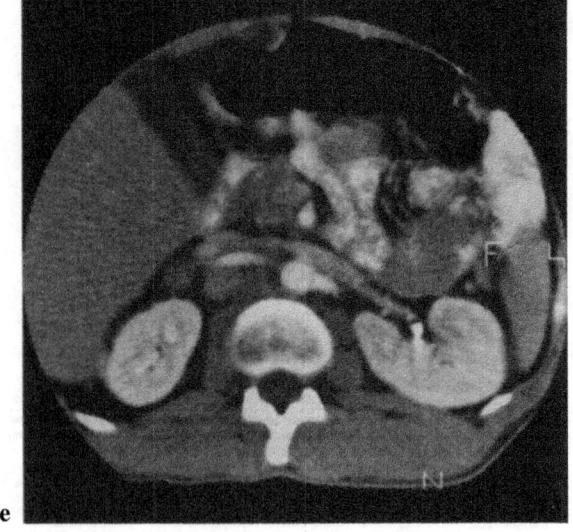

e

Inj. **81**

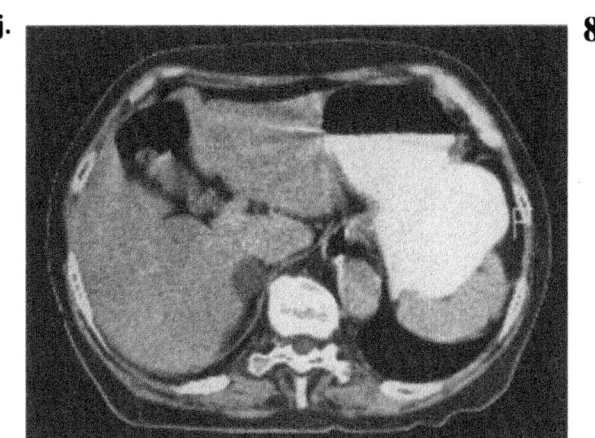

Inj. **82**

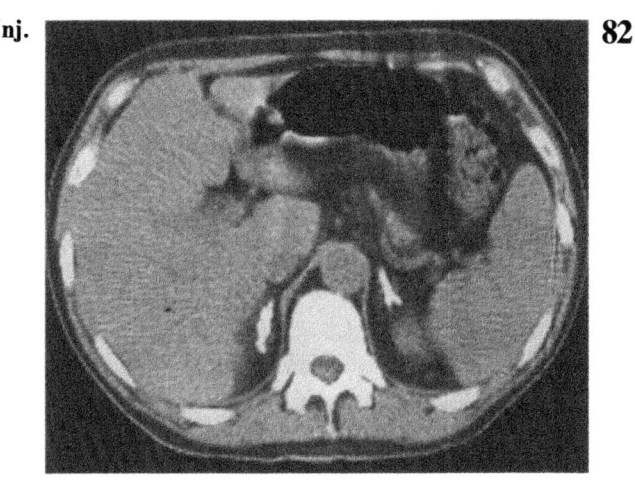

83

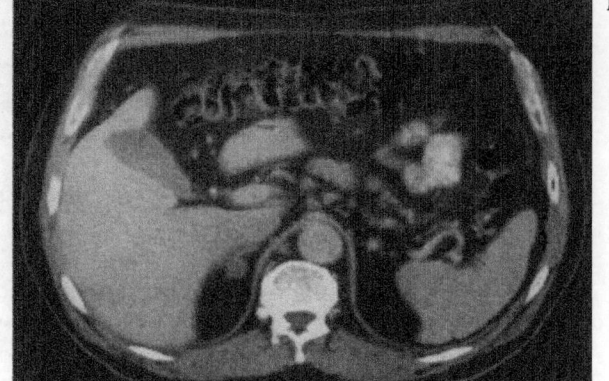

Inj.

a

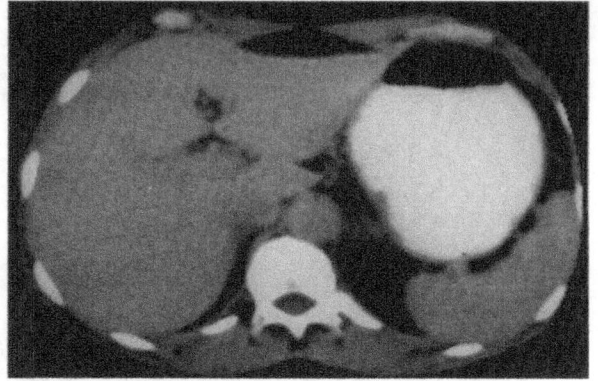

Inj.

b

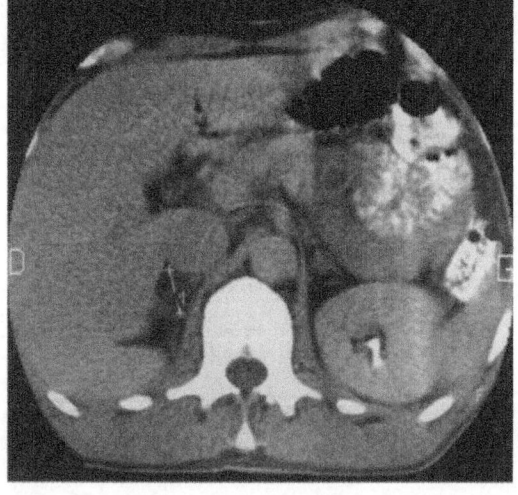

Inj.

c

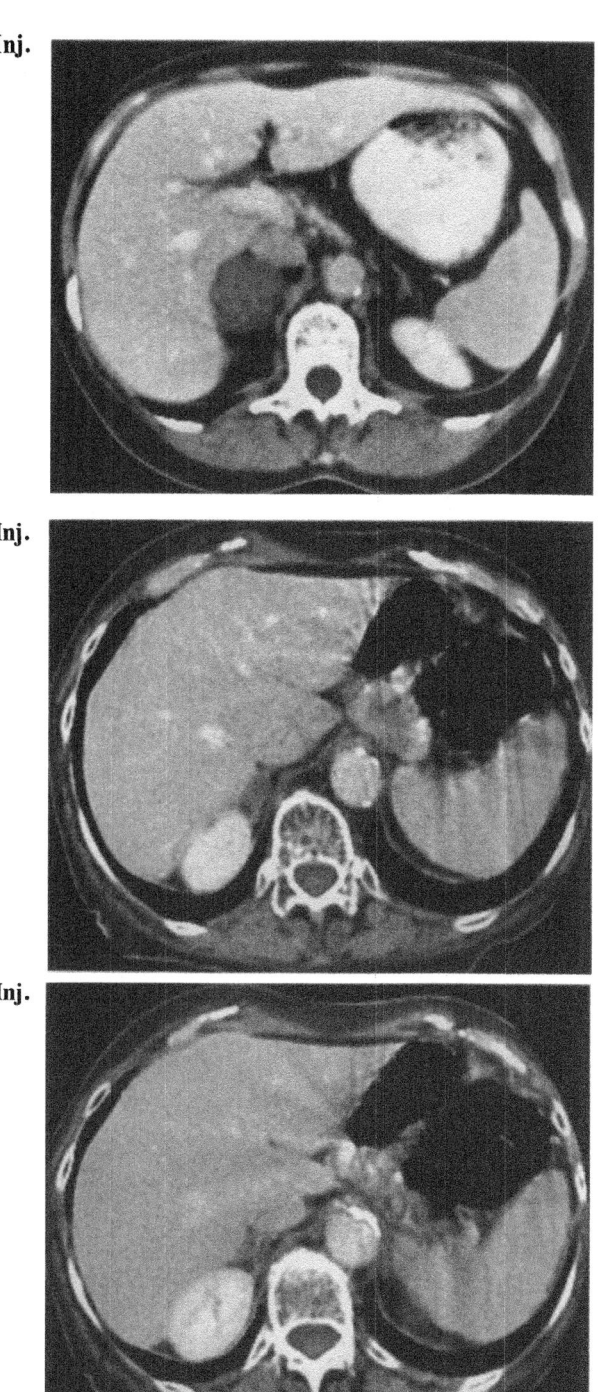

83

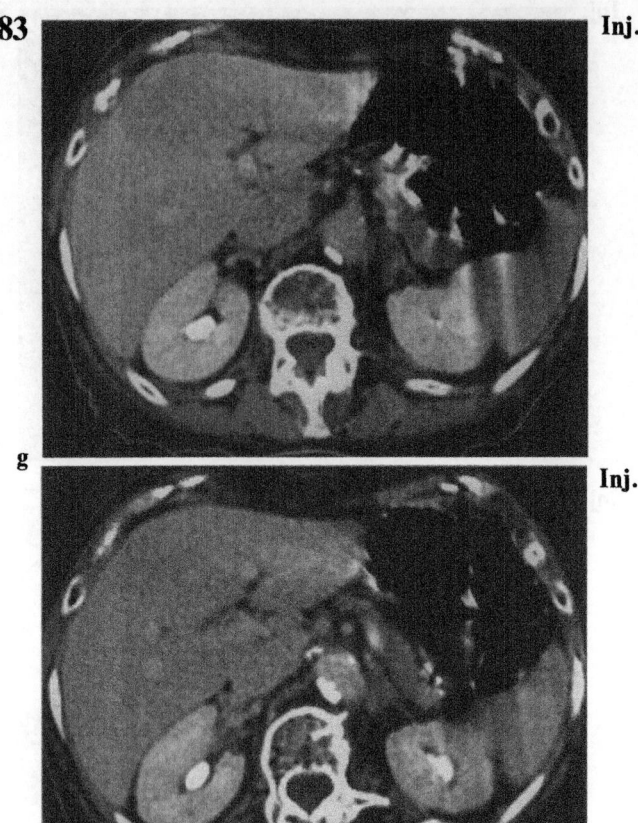

g

h

Inj.

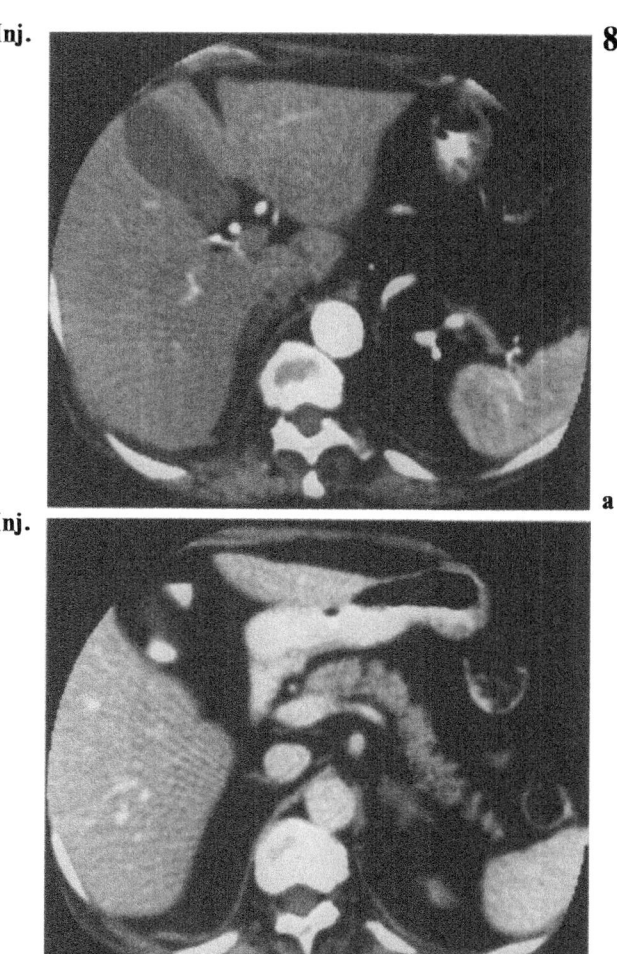

a

Inj.

b

84

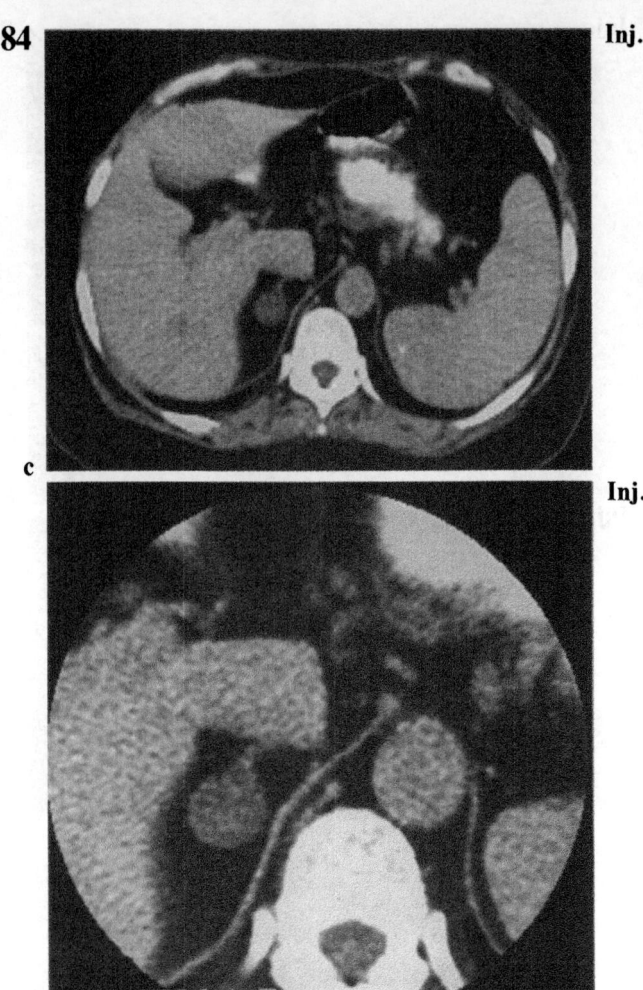

c

FONCTION ?

d

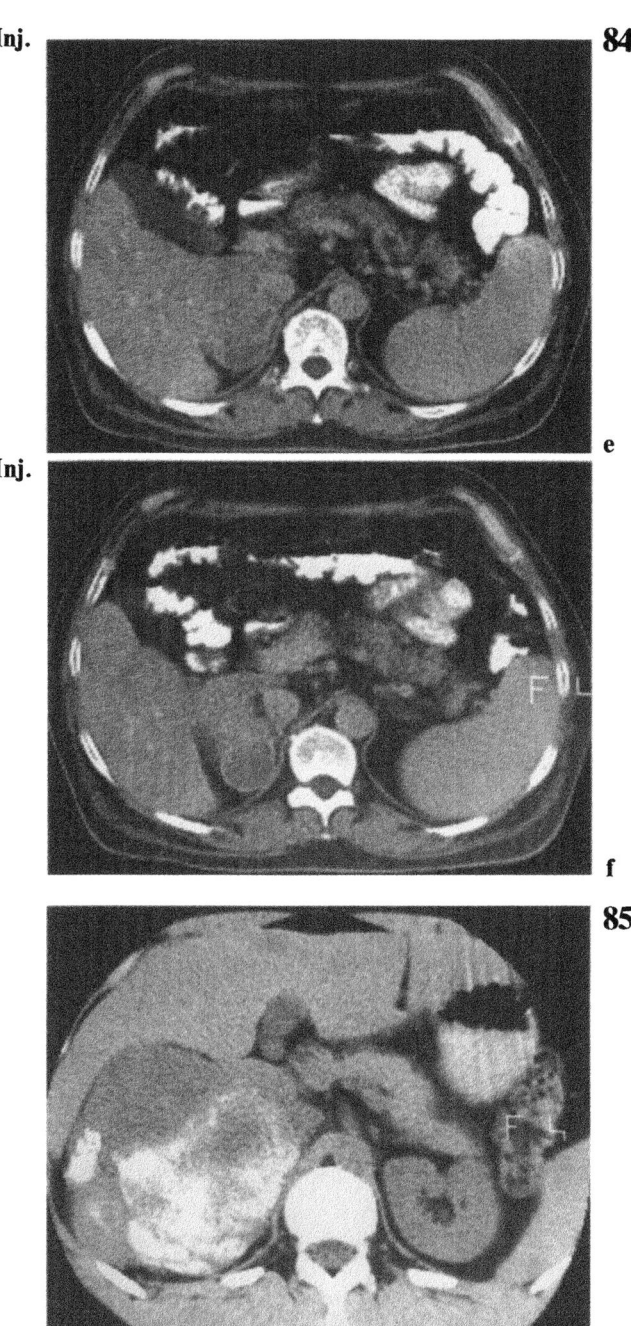

Part Two

Commentary with Corresponding Schemata

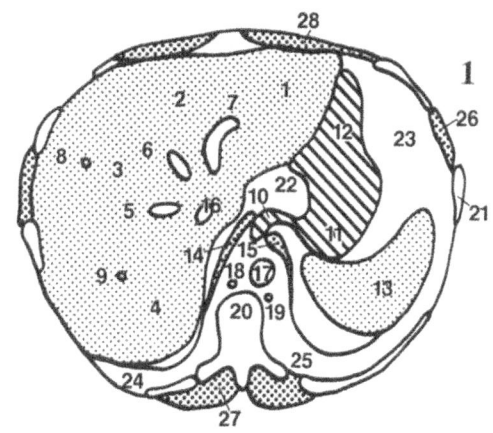

1 segment II
2 segment IV
3 segment VIII
4 segment VII
5 Right hepatic vein
6 Middle hepatic vein
7 Left hepatic vein
8 Anterior branch of the right branch of the portal vein
9 Posterior branch of the right branch of the portal vein
10 Cardia
11 Greater curvature
12 Fundus
13 Spleen
14 Right crus of diaphragm
15 Left crus of diaphragm
16 Inferior vena cava
17 Aorta
18 Vena azygos
19 Vena hemiazygos
20 Vertebral body of T11
21 Ribs

22 Lesser omentum
23 Greater peritoneal sac
24 Inferior lobe of the right lung
25 Inferior lobe of the left lung
26 Intercostal muscles
27 Spinal muscles
28 Rectus abdominis muscle

Segment I has not been omitted; it will be displayed in figure 2.

This slice passes through the hepatic dome and through the upper vertebral body of T11 (20) (section plane 1). At this level the thoracic part of the esophagus passes through the diaphragm (14, 15) and becomes the abdominal part, to end at the cardiac orifice of the stomach (10). The posterior inframediastinal space is occupied by the aorta (17) and the azygos vessels (18, 19). The thoracic duct is not visible; this can be demonstrated only with lymphography.

The most important organ at this level is the liver. The three hepatic veins (5–7) are readily recognizable with their longitudinal section since they have here a horizontal course; they radiate from a center constituted by the inferior vena cava (16).

The middle hepatic vein (6) separates the right part of the liver (3, 4) from the left part (1, 2), according to a plane indicated on the section by a line joining the middle hepatic vein with the inferior vena cava. The right (5) and the left (7) hepatic veins are intersegmental. The right hepatic vein separates the anterior segment (3) from the posterior segment (4) of the right part of the liver; the left hepatic vein separates the lateral segment (1) from the median segment (2) of the left part of the liver. This slice also shows the anterior (8) and posterior (9) branches of the right branch of the portal vein sectioned transversely, since they have here a vertical course.

At the level of the hepatic convexity, the following segments are seen:
– Lateral segment or segment II (1)
– Median segment or segment IV (2)
– Anterior segment or segment VIII (3)
– Posterior segment or segment VII (4)

2

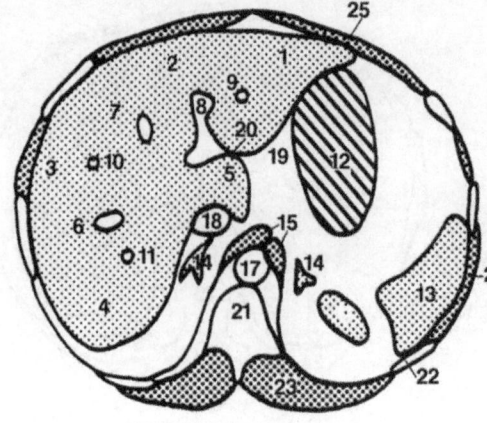

1 Lateral segment = segment II + III
2 Median segment = segment IV
3 Anterior segment = segment V + VIII
4 Posterior segment = segment VI + VII
5 Caudate lobe = segment I
6 Right hepatic vein
7 Middle hepatic vein
8 Left branch of the portal vein in the fissure for the round ligament of the liver
9 Portal branch for segment II

10 Anterior branch of the right branch of the portal vein
11 Posterior branch of the right branch of the portal vein
12 Stomach
13 Spleen
14 Adrenal gland
15 Crus of diaphragm
16 Left kidney
17 Aorta
18 Inferior vena cava
19 Lesser omentum
20 Arantius canal
21 Vertebral body of T11
22 Rib
23 Spinal muscles
24 Intercostal muscles
25 Rectus abdominis muscle

This slice passes above the porta hepatis and through the vertebral body of T11 (*21*) (section plane 2).

As in the previous slice, the middle hepatic vein (*7*) separates the right from the left part of the liver. Since this vein now has a vertical course, its appearance differs: it is here sectioned transversely and appears as a circular structure. The same is true for the right hepatic vein (*6*), which still separates the anterior (*3*) from the posterior (*4*) segment of the right part of the liver.

On the left the hepatic vein is no longer visible, but the left branch of the portal vein (*8*) becomes the landmark which separates segment IV (*2*) and segments II and III (*1*) in the left part of the liver. After the porta hepatis the left branch first has a vertical course (as we shall see on the following slice) and then curves forward with an anteroposterior horizontal course in the fissure for the round ligament of the liver (*8*). The latter is well visible in this slice. At this level the left branch gives off a branch (*9*) for segment II.

The anterior (*10*) and the posterior (*11*) branches of the right branch of the portal vein are seen between the intersegmental hepatic veins. At this level one can see the caudate lobe or segment I (*5*), bound dorsally by the inferior vena cava (*18*) and ventrally by Arantius' canal (*20*).

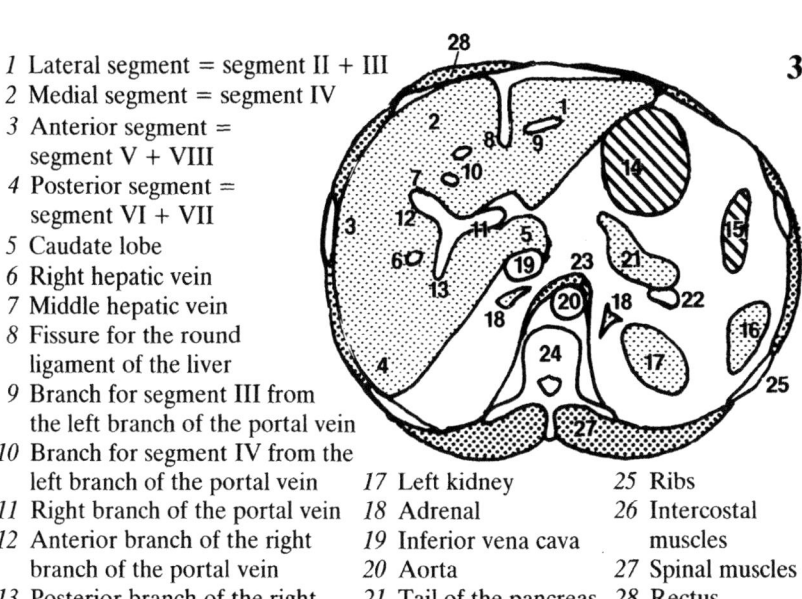

1 Lateral segment = segment II + III
2 Medial segment = segment IV
3 Anterior segment = segment V + VIII
4 Posterior segment = segment VI + VII
5 Caudate lobe
6 Right hepatic vein
7 Middle hepatic vein
8 Fissure for the round ligament of the liver
9 Branch for segment III from the left branch of the portal vein
10 Branch for segment IV from the left branch of the portal vein
11 Right branch of the portal vein
12 Anterior branch of the right branch of the portal vein
13 Posterior branch of the right branch of the portal vein
14 Stomach (fundus)
15 Left colic flexure
16 Spleen

17 Left kidney
18 Adrenal
19 Inferior vena cava
20 Aorta
21 Tail of the pancreas
22 Splenic artery
23 Crus of diaphragm
24 Vertebral body of T12

25 Ribs
26 Intercostal muscles
27 Spinal muscles
28 Rectus abdominis

This slice passes through the porta hepatis and the upper plate of the 12th thoracic vertebra (*24*) (section plane 3). The middle hepatic vein (*7*) separates the right part of the liver (*3, 4*) from the left part (*1, 2*). The right hepatic vein (*6*) still separates the anterior segment (*3*) from the posterior segment (*4*) of the right liver. As in the previous slice, the left hepatic vein is not visible at this level. The fissure for the round ligament of the liver (*8*) separates the lateral segment (*1*) from the medial segment (*2*) of the left liver. This slice is of interest since it displays the right branch of the portal vein (*11*) as well as its anterior (*12*) and posterior (*13*) division branches, which have a horizontal course and are thus seen in longitudinal section.

The anterior branch (*12*) for the anterior segment and the posterior branch (*13*) for the posterior segment of the right liver form an angle containing the right hepatic vein (*6*).

The caudate lobe is situated between the portal vein in front and the inferior vena cava behind; it has direct drainage into the inferior vena cava and receives directly the portal vessels from either the left or the right branch or from both.

At this level the tip of the spleen (*16*) and the fundus (*14*) are still visible and there appear:

– The left colic flexure (*15*)
– The tail of the pancreas (*21*) with the loops of the splenic artery (*22*)
– The adrenal (*18*)
– The upper pole of the left kidney (*17*)

4

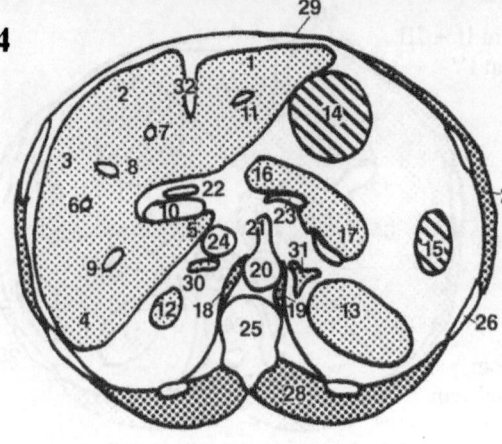

10 Portal vein
11 Branch of the left branch of the portal vein for the d nage of the lateral segment
12 Right kidney
13 Left kidney
14 Stomach
15 Descending colon
16 Body of the pancreas
17 Tail of the pancreas
18 Right crus of the diaphragm
19 Left crus of the diaphragm
20 Aorta
21 Celiac trunk
22 Hepatic artery
23 Splenic artery
24 Inferior vena cava
25 Vertebral body of T12
26 Ribs
27 Intercostal muscles
28 Spinal muscles
29 Rectus abdominis
30 Right adrenal gland
31 Left adrenal gland
32 Fissure for round ligament of the liver

1 Lateral segment = segment III
2 Medial segment = segment IV
3 Anterior segment = segment V
4 Posterior segment = segment VI
5 Caudate lobe
6 Right hepatic vein
7 Middle hepatic vein
8 Anterior branch of the right branch of the portal vein
9 Posterior branch of the right branch of the portal vein

This slice passes below the porta hepatis, through the body (*16*) and the tail (*17*) of the pancreas, and through the lower vertebral plate of the 12th thoracic vertebra (*25*) (section plane 4). The hepatic segmentation remains the same: the middle hepatic vein (*7*) separates the left liver (*1, 2*) from the right liver (*3, 4*), the right hepatic vein (*6*) separates the anterior segment or segment V (*3*) from the posterior segment or segment VI (*4*), and, finally, the fissure for the round ligament or ligamentum teres (*32*) marks the limit between the lateral segment or segment III (*1*) and the median segment or segment IV (*2*). The caudate lobe (*5*) is represented only by a thin layer of parenchyma bound ventrally by the portal vein (*10*) and dorsally by the inferior vena cava (*24*).

The aorta (*20*) gives rise to the celiac trunk (*21*) whose two main branches are visible:
1. the hepatic artery (*22*) sectioned transversely anterior to the portal vein (*10*)
2. the splenic artery (*23*), well visualized longitudinally posterior to the body and the tail of the pancreas (*16, 17*).

Other structures displayed include the stomach (*14*), descending colon (*15*), right (*18*) and left (*19*) crus of the diaphragm, adrenals (*30, 31*), and kidneys (*12, 13*).

1 Right part of the liver
2 Gallbladder
3 Descending part of the duodenum
4 Jejunal loops
5 Transverse colon
6 Descending colon
7 Head of the pancreas
8 Abdominal aorta
9 Inferior vena cava
10 Superior mesenteric artery
11 Superior mesenteric vein
12 Left renal artery
13 Left renal vein
14 Insertion of right crus of diaphragm
15 Right and left kidneys
16 Vertebral body of L1

17 Ribs
18 Spinal muscles
19 Intercostal muscles
20 Rectus abdominis

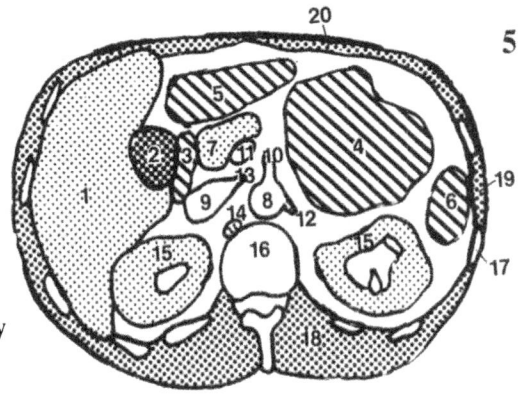

This slice passes through the head of the pancreas (7) and the first lumbar vertebra (16) (section plane 5). The head of the pancreas is easily recognizable because it is always framed by constant structures: on the right by the descending part of the duodenum (3) (especially as it is opacified) and on the left and behind by the superior mesenteric vessels – the superior mesenteric vein (11) on the right within the pancreatic parenchyma, and the superior mesenteric artery (10) more to the left, where it arises from the abdominal aorta (8).

A rounded hypodensity, 3–5 mm in diameter and corresponding to the choledochus is often visualized on the posterior and right part of the pancreatic head (7).

The gallbladder (2) is well defined with its liquid-type densities and its thin (1- to 2-mm-thick) wall, but this does not serve as a landmark. Although it is usually located in the interlobar fissure, its situation is variable.

The stomach is no longer visible; there appear the jejunal loops (4), more or less opacified, and more laterally and to the left, the descending colon (6). Both kidneys (15) are now well displayed, with the surrounding parenchyma and the opacified calyceal cavities in the center. Note also the slightly too-high arising of the left renal artery (12).

6

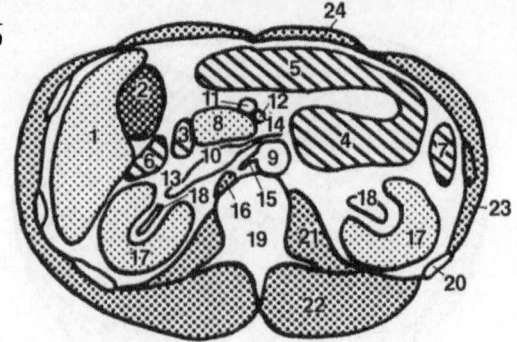

1 Right liver lobe	*10* Inferior vena cava	*20* Ribs
2 Gallbladder	*11* Superior mesenteric vein	*21* Psoas muscles
3 Descending part	*12* Superior mesenteric artery	*22* Spinal muscles
of the duodenum	*13* Right renal vein	*23* Intercostal muscles
4 Jejunal loops	*14* Left renal vein	*24* Rectus abdominis
5 Transverse colon	*15* Right renal artery	muscle
6 Descending colon	*16* Right crus of the diaphragm	
7 Ascending colon	*17* Left and right kidneys	
8 Winslow's pancreas	*18* Renal pelvis	
9 Aorta	*19* Vertebral body of L2	

This slice passes through Winslow's pancreas (*8*), the hilus renalis (*17*) and the second lumbar vertebra (*19*) (section plane 6).

Like the pancreatic head, the uncinate process of the pancreas (*8*) is delimited by constant structures: on the right by the descending part of the duodenum (*3*), and on the left and anteriorly by the superior mesenteric vessels; the vein (*11*), larger than the artery (*12*), is situated on its right.

Following intravenous contrast-medium administration, only the renal pelvis remains opacified in the renal hilum.

The course of the vessels is demonstrated, especially for the veins, which are larger than the arteries. The right renal vein (*13*) has a short course from the inferior vena cava (*10*) to the renal hilum. It lies in front of and slightly above the right renal artery (*15*).

However the right renal artery has a long retrocaval course. It is usually thinner than the vein (*13*) and is rarely visible in its full length.

The left renal vein (*14*) has also a long course between the aorta (*9*) and the mesenteric artery (*12*), which runs above and then in front of it. The passage through the mesentericoaortic clip may be responsible for the decreased caliber of the vein, without this having pathologic significance. The left renal artery has a short course and is usually visible only at its origin on the aorta. It is seen behind and slightly below the homolateral renal vein. The insertion of the right crus of the diaphragm (*16*) must not be mistaken for adenopathy.

The psoas muscles (*21*) appear in this slice.

100

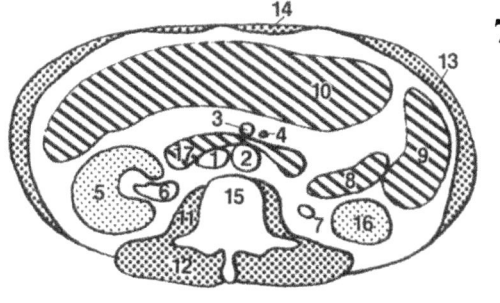

7

1 Inferior vena cava
2 Abdominal aorta
3 Superior mesenteric vein
4 Superior mesenteric artery
5 Right kidney
6 Right renal pelvis
7 Left ureter
8 Small intestine loops
9 Descending colon
10 Digestive tract
11 Psoas muscles
12 Spinal muscles
13 Transverse muscles, external
   and internal oblique muscles

14 Rectus abdominis
15 Vertebral body of L3
16 Left kidney
17 Horizontal or third part of the duodenum

This slice passes through the horizontal part of the duodenum (*17*) and the third lumbar vertebra (*15*) (section plane 7).

At this level the horizontal part of the duodenum (*17*) is related to the inferior surface of the pancreas. The right renal pelvis (*6*) is still visible at this level. It appears as an oblong cavity of liquid-type density before the administration of iodine or hyperdense after contrast administration, as shown here.

On the left, the section already passes below the renal hilus and shows the left ureter (*7*), when it is opacified, as a white point in front of and lateral to the psoas muscles (*11*). The digestive tract (*10*) – loops of the small intestine (*8*), descending colon (*9*), mesentery, and greater omentum–occupy the peritoneal cavity.

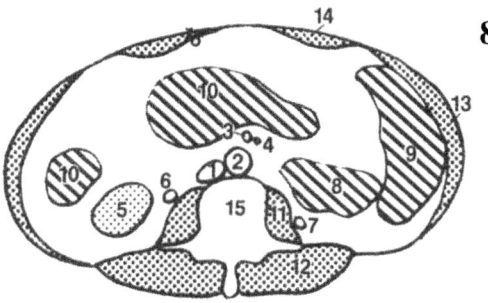

8

1 Inferior vena cava
2 Aorta
3 Superior mesenteric vein
4 Superior mesenteric artery
5 Right kidney
6 Right ureter
7 Left ureter
8 Loops of small intestine
9 Descending colon
10 Digestive tract
11 Psoas muscles
12 Spinal muscles
13 Transverse muscles, external and
   internal oblique muscles

14 Rectus abdominis
15 L3/4 disk

This slice passes through the lower pole of the right kidney and through the L3/4 disk (section plane 8).
It differs from the previous one only by:
– Absence of the left kidney and of the horizontal part of the duodenum
– Presence of the ureter in the prolongation of the renal pelvis
The contents of the abdominal cavity are identical.

9

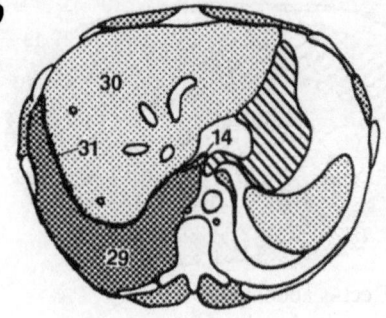 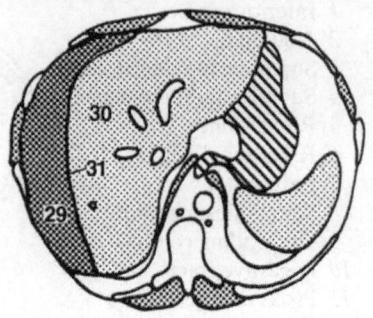

The diagnosis of ascites and of pleural effusion should not prove difficult here. Two signs allow the differentiation of these conditions:
1. Location of the crus of the diaphragm with regard to the effusion. The crus lies in front of the pleural effusion and behind ascites.
2. The interface of liquid to liver or spleen is ill-defined in pleural effusion but well-defined with ascites. Interposition of the diaphragm between the liver and pleural effusion accounts for the lack of clarity, while its absence renders the interface very clear.

Scan **9a** corresponds to section level 1 (p. 95). The crus of the diaphragm (*14*) lies anterior to the effusion (*29*), which hints at pleural location. The interface (*31*) of effusion (*29*) to liver (*30*) is ill-defined, which also suggests pleural location.

Now, study also scan **9c**: What is the etiology of this pleural effusion (**a** and **c**)? We note that this patient has hepatic (*30*) and bony (*20*) lesions: metastases from breast cancer.

Scan **9b** also corresponds to section level 1 (p. 95).

The right crus of the diaphragm (*14*) is seen between the liver (*30*) and the air-containing pleural recess (*32*). The boundary (*31*) between fluid (*29*) and liver (*30*) is well-defined on the entire hepatic contour. This is ascites, as confirmed by **d**.

These three scans show the typical computerized tomographic (CT) appearance of a rare but severe disease: Budd-Chiari's syndrome. **10**

Scan **10a** (section level 2, p. 96): This plain scan demonstrates well hepatomegaly and hypertrophy of the caudate lobe (5) as well as the contrast between the density of the periphery and that of the center of the liver.

Scan **10b**: Injection of iodine increases the differential contrast between the periphery, which remains hypodense, and the center, which shows nonhomogeneous uptake of contrast. The hepatic veins are not demonstrated; they are said to be "excluded." The delayed scan **10c** shows partial uptake of contrast in the peripheral segments due to fibrosis. The areas which remain hypodense are necrotic.

3 Heart **11**
4 Esophagus
5 Aorta
6 Pleural recess
7 T10

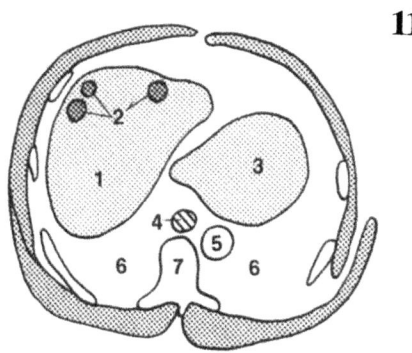

This section was taken in the very upper part of the liver (*1*). Echography of the liver had shown several rounded, echo-free areas. CT scans confirm the diagnosis of multiple, small, benign cysts (*2*).

These lesions have, in fact, all the characteristics of benign cysts:
– Rounded, oval lesions or lobulated in the case of multilocular cysts
– Liquid density (0–15 HU)
– Thin and smooth walls
– No septations
– No preferential location
– Usually no calcification
– No changes after contrast injection

The density of the cyst can also be higher, for instance, when there is infection or hemorrhage; it may also be due to a partial-volume phenomenon when the cyst is small.

12

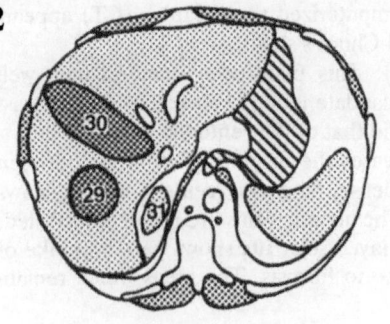

This hepatic lesion (*29*) is single and has a diameter of 3.5 cm. This scanography was performed because the patient complained of abdominal pain; it shows another appearance of a benign cyst.

The criteria enumerated previously are all present here, but note also:
– Number: from one to several cysts
– Size: variable, ranging from 1 mm to several centimeters in diameter

To comment upon this image, we need to refer to section level 1, p. 95, taking into account that the present scan was taken with the patient in deep inspiration. This accounts for the fact that the gallbladder (*30*) and the right kidney (*31*) are already visible.

On the basis of these data, the diagnosis of benign cyst is easy. When the wall is slightly thickened or irregular, or when there is a septum, one must consider the presence of an abscess, of a long-standing hematoma, or, more rarely, of a necrotic malignant tumor. Needle biopsy may be helpful for this diagnosis.

A very large number of cysts suggests the presence of polycystosis and should lead one to search for cysts in the kidneys and in the pancreas.

13

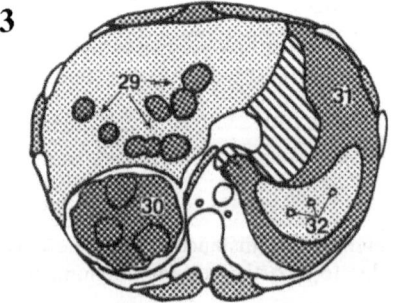

The presence of numerous hepatic cysts (*29*) in this patient with hepato-renal polycystosis leads to the search for renal lesions (*30*) (section level 1, p. 95).

Note also the presence of trivial calcifications of the spleen (*32*) and of retroperitoneal effusion (*31*). This patient suffers from renal failure and is treated by peritoneal dialysis.

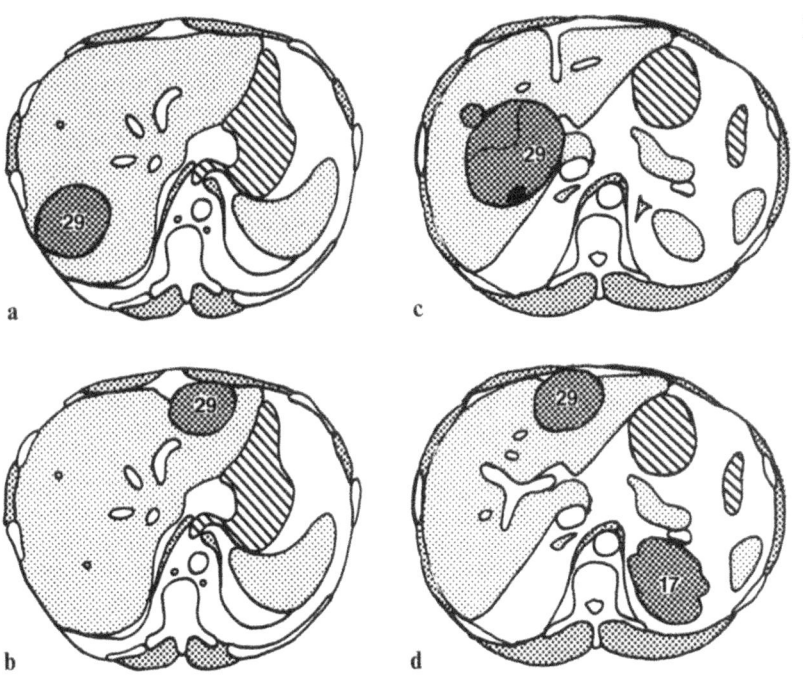

These four images of cystic diseases of the liver illustrate certain appearances of hepatic masses with liquid density.

a: Parasitic cyst. This lesion (*29*) of the right liver lobe possesses almost all the characteristics of a biliary cyst, except for too-thick walls (section level 1, p. 95). A history of colic amebiasis and positive serology permit the diagnosis of amebic abscess of the liver (cf. scans 15, 16).

b: Subcapsular hematoma (cf. scan 39). Only the history of trauma to the right hypochondrium and of subcapsular effusion diagnosed from ultrasonography 6 weeks earlier allow one to conclude subcapsular hematoma (*29*) of the liver (section level 1, p. 95).

c: Hepatoma (cf. scans 25–28). This is a multiple hepatoma, the main lesion of which (*29*), although mainly cystic, shows septations and a parietal tumoral mass (section level 3, p. 97).

d: Biliary cyst (*29*) (cf. scans 11, 12). The liquid-type lesions in the left lumbar region correspond to simple cysts (cf. cases 64, 65) of the upper pole of the left kidney (*17*) (section level 3, p. 97).

15

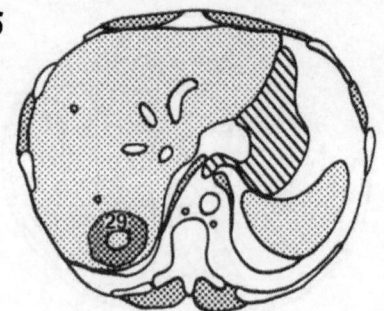

This section was performed in the upper part of the liver before intravenous contrast injection (section level 1, p. 95). There is a rounded lesion, 7 cm in diameter (*29*) in the posterior part of the right liver lobe (more precisely, in segment VII), with a density between that of a cyst and that of a solid tumor – isodense in the center and hypodense in the periphery.

Diagnostic hypotheses here would be premature. At this stage of the investigation and in the absence of clinical data it is impossible to indicate an etiology, for one would have to enumerate all focal lesions of the liver (cyst, abscess, tumor, malformations, etc.). Now proceed to scan 16.

16 This scan is taken in the same patient as in scan 15 after intravenous injection of contrast medium. Two changes must be noted:
- Enhancement of the hepatic parenchyma
- Appearance of an anular contrast uptake at the periphery of the lesion

This reaction to iodine injection permits us to rule out:
- Benign cyst, which never takes up contrast
- Benign tumors, especially hemangiomas, whose characteristic response to contrast will be shown in another case (i.e., centripetal opacification)

There remain two etiologies to be considered, abscess and malignant tumors. The presence of an amebic abscess is suggested here by the clinical context:
- History of colic amebiasis 25 years previously
- Pain in the right hypochondrium
- Temperature of 39° for 10 days
This diagnosis was confirmed by the serology.

A closer view allows one to point out the CT characteristics of an abscess:
- A rounded mass, of variable size, usually single
- Density between that of cyst and that of solid tumor before iodine injection
- Walls with a thickness of several millimeters, clear external contours, and occasionally irregular internal contours; these are clearly enhanced after intravenous contrast injection
- No change in the density of contents following intravenous injection; this is an important sign, since central enhancement suggests neoplastic or inflammatory etiology rather than an abscess
- The preferential site is the posterior part of the right liver
- Spontaneous presence of air in 20%–30% of the cases, excepting amebic abscesses which never contain air unless there has been a rupture into the digestive cavity or puncture

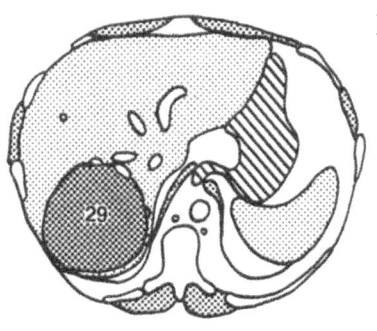

This image suggests only one diagnosis: hydatid cyst (*29*).

Let us consider this pathognomonic image however in more detail. The diagnosis is consistent with the following features:

- A uni- or multilocular mass
- Its density is of the fluid type
- Its wall is thin and smooth and enhanced after contrast injection
- There are rounded or oval microcysts (*29*) within the cyst which have more or less thick walls
- There are numerous parietal linear calcifications

Together, these five criteria allow the diagnosis of hydatid cyst, i.e., a multilocular cyst with thin walls, enhanced by contrast injection or calcified and containing daughter cells with septae of variable thickness (section level 1, p. 95).

18

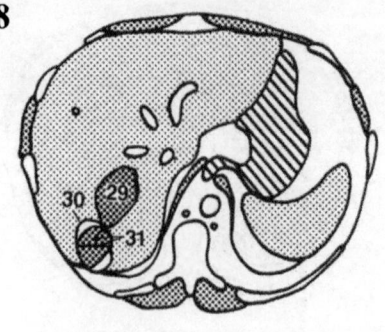

These two scans illustrate a less characteristic appearance of granular hydatidosis.

Scan **a** passes through the hepatic dome and shows a homogeneous, discretely lobulated, noncalcified structure with a density of about +30 HU (*29*).

Hydatid cysts usually have densities of a fluid, i.e., between 0 and +15 HU, however higher values may occur (up to + 40 HU), as may also much lower values (−200 to −500 HU), reflecting the presence of air following superinfection or rupture into a digestive structure.

Scan **b**: Whereas scan **a** alone is not conclusive, this one represents a more caudal slice and shows a more specific image of a cyst, with calcified walls (*30*) and internal septations (*31*). The diagnosis, confirmed by biological measurements, is hydatid cyst (section level 1, p. 95).

19

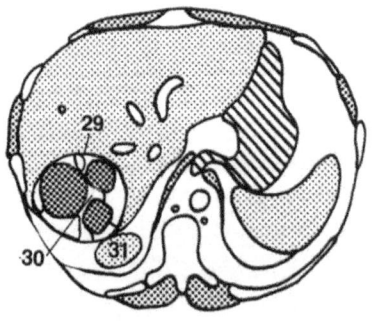

31 Right kidney

This scan shows another CT appearance of hydatid cyst. The parietal calcifications (*29*) can be thicker and more irregular, and the contents themselves may undergo calcification due to deposits (*30*), especially in longstanding cysts (section level 1, p. 95).

Before ending this series on atypical hydatid cysts, we should point out that a unique, noncalcified mass showing the density of a fluid may hide a hydatid cyst. When there is doubt, serology will confirm or falsify the diagnosis.

These two scans were taken before and after injection of contrast medium in the same patient (section level 4, p. 98) and should be analyzed successively:

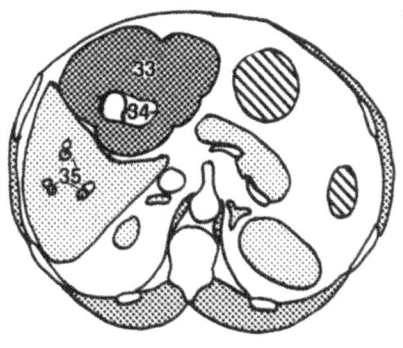

- There is a circumscribed lesion in the left part of the liver (*33*) (segments II, III, and IV); it is heterogeneous, globally hypodense between +15 and +40 HU
- It contains numerous, clustered, small calcifications (*34*)
- The lesion involves the porta hepatis and perhaps the caudate lobe
- Densities are unchanged after contrast injection
- The intrahepatic bile ducts (*35*) in the normal parenchyma are dilated; these are seen as rounded structures with a diameter of several millimeters and fluid densities around each portal vessel

When there is such a lesion, four main diagnoses should be considered:
- hepatocellular carcinoma
- metastasis
- alveolar hydatidosis
- granular hydatidosis

This is, in fact, a case of alveolar echinococcosis, as was confirmed by the specific determination of the antigen by immunoelectrophoresis.

Which of our findings suggest this etiology that, although rare, should not be mistaken? First of all, there are the five signs described above as specific to alveolar echinococcosis.

Calcifications are present in 80%–90% of the cases. These consist of polycyclic microcalcifications, which are quite different from the larger, irregular, disseminated calcifications seen in hepatomas and in parietal calcifications of the hydatid cysts.

Like metastases, the hepatoma is enhanced after contrast injection.

Moreover, in hepatomas, metastases, and hydatid cysts there is usually no dilatation of the intrahepatic bile ducts in the normal parenchyma.

Finally, there are the clinical and the biological data, namely:
- Hard and painful hepatic tumor
- Alteration of the general status
- Hypereosinophilia
- Anicteric cholestasis
- Hypergammaglobulinemia of IgM

21

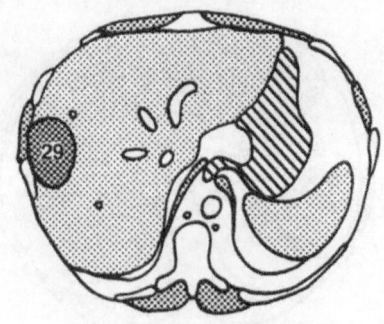

If, regarding this scan taken prior to contrast injection, one were asked to make a single diagnosis, one would be correct in refusing to do so; radiology, after all, is not a riddle.

Nevertheless, I persist with my question, for it is very often necessary to know what one is looking for in order to find it.

This hypodense mass (*29*), which is discretely lobulated, oval with a long diameter of 4 cm, homogeneous, and well demarcated, suggests first of all a benign tumor of the liver and, then, in order of declining frequency of occurrence, hemangioma, adenoma, focal nodular hyperplasia, and primary or secondary maligant tumor.

Upon learning, then, that this case is one of a 50-year-old woman without particular antecedents, one should consider immediately the possibility of a benign tumor, in particular a hemangioma, since this is the most frequent benign tumor of the liver (3%–7% of the population and clearly predominant in females).

The diagnosis of a hemangioma requires a peculiar technique, with images taken at precise intervals after injection:
– First image at 30 s
– Second image between 2 and 4 min
– Third, delayed image at 8–10 min

This method gives evidence of the almost pathognomonic behavior of a hemangioma (*29*) (section level 1, p. 95).

As seen in scan 22, the three parts of which were taken are intervals as described above.

22 Scan **a**, taken 30 s after contrast-medium administration, demonstrates early and intense enhancement of a part of the periphery of the lesion.

In some cases intense enhancement occurs in the entire periphery of the lesion.

b, performed 3 min after contrast injection, shows total and intense opacification of the lesion. Note that opacification is centripetal: it goes from the periphery to the center. This is quasi-pathognomonic of the behavior of hemangiomas.

c, finally, taken 5 min after contrast injection, demonstrates the persistence of opacification, which is not the case with adenomas, hyperplasia, and metastases.

Before proceeding, I would like to point out some general characteristics of cavernous hemangiomas. We consider here only the cavernous hemangioma with a diameter between 2.5 and 5 cm; hemangiomas with a diameter under 2 cm raise diagnostic problems which are dealt with below, and hemangiomas with a diameter above 5 cm are rare.

This solid benign tumor is rounded or lobulated, homogeneous, and hypodense before injection; it has clearly defined margins. It is isolated, rarely calcified, and often infracapsular. It is encountered most frequently in older women (70% of the cases) and is asymptomatic. Its behavior after contrast injection is characteristic (provided that images are made early and are then repeated at regular intervals): intense and early peripheral enhancement, centripetal progression, and delayed persistence of contrast.

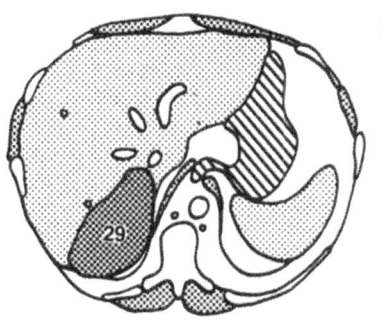

23

Is it necessary to point out that these four images have been performed on the same patient, at the same level, in four very precise phases (before injection, 30 s, 3 min, and 10 min after injection) in order to make the diagnosis of cavernous hemangioma (*29*) (section level 1, p. 95)?

Note the peculiarities in each.

a shows a more marked, central hypodensity (*29*); this indicates partial thrombosis of the hemangioma, a frequent occurrence when there is a large mass (here the hemangioma has a diameter of 5 cm). Note also the presence of a benign cyst in the extremity of the left lobe.

b demonstrates an almost circumferential, early, and intense enhancement.

c shows the centripetal progression.

d does not display the total opacification; this is frequent with large-sized hemangiomas, which are often the site of partial central thrombosis.

24

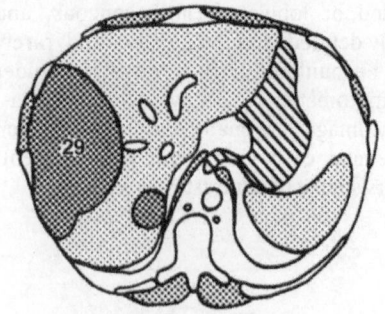

These images (section level 1, p. 95), performed on a 40-year-old woman complaining of abdominal pain indicate multiple hemangiomas.

This case, however, is remarkable for:
- Multiplicity of the lesions: two
- Size of the lesions: 7.5 cm and 3.5 cm (*29*)

As has already been pointed out, hemangiomas are generally single and are rarely above 5 cm in size.

As is the case with most large hemangiomas, we note here the absence of total, delayed opacification.

25

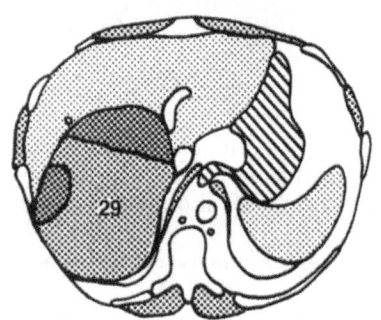

These scans have been performed before and after contrast injection; they display the most common malignant primary tumor of the liver – solitary hepatoma (section level 1, p. 95):

- Voluminous mass (*29*) (usually with a diameter greater than 2.5 cm) causing deformation of the liver contour
- Hypodense with regard to the normal parenchyma
- More or less irregular limits
- Heterogeneous opacification, beginning at the periphery following bolus injection

Besides these criteria, which are always present and already suggest a neoplasm, other signs indicating a malignant process must be sought:
- Vascular involvement, which appears as a lacunar image within the vascular lumen (portal or hepatic) following contrast injection; thrombosis of a portal branch can be accompanied by necrosis – this feature is more important than the size of the tumor, since it affects a vascular territory (also comprising normal parenchyma)
- Increased caliber of the hepatic artery
- Arteriovenous shunt with simultaneous visualization of the aorta and the portal vein on an image taken during bolus injection
- Locoregional extension, adenopathies, and ascites

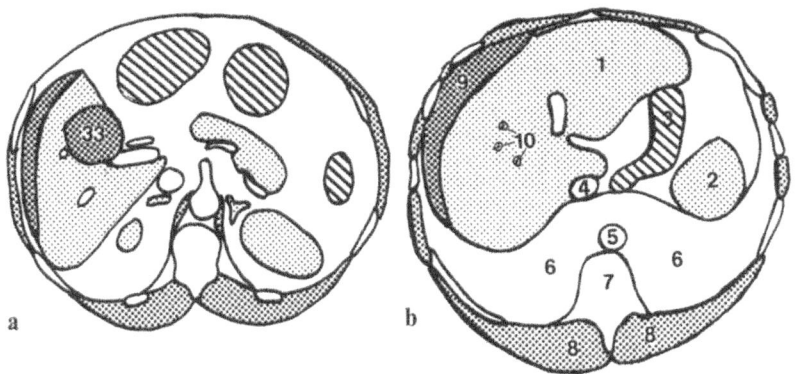

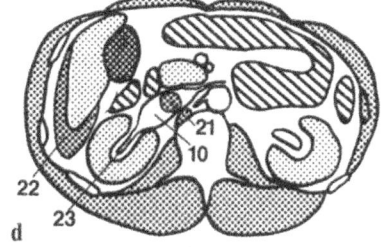

1 Liver
2 Spleen
3 Stomach
4 Inferior vena cava
5 Aorta
6 Pleural sinus
7 Thoracic spine
8 Spinal muscles
9 Ascites
10 Dilated bile ducts

These two cases, a, b and c, d, illustrate two pecularities of hepatomas, related respectively to their location and to their aggressivity.

a (section level 4, p. 98): A tumor of the porta hepatis (*33*). This location results rapidly in dilatation of the intrahepatic bile ducts (better demonstrated in **b**).

c: The tumor involving segments VII and VIII of the liver is complicated by parietal invasion and by a quite uncommon vascular involvement, namely extension to the inferior vena cava.

d (section level 6, p. 100): This involvement (*21*) is well visible as a hypodensity within the enlarged inferior vena cava (*10*). *22* Ascites, *23* Right renal vein

27

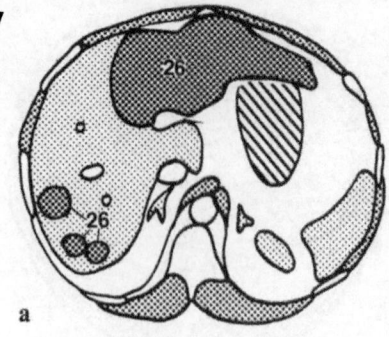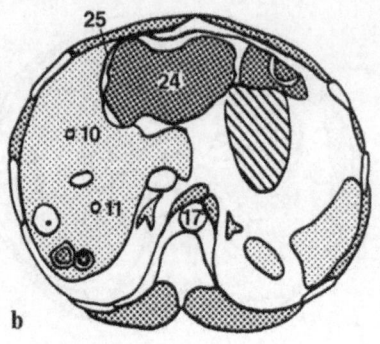

a

b

Scan **a**, taken prior to injection, shows several hypodense areas (26) in the hepatic parenchyma which correspond to a multifocal hepatoma, another appearance of hepatomas (section level 2, p. 96).

b and **c**, taken immediately after bolus injection, show two signs specific to hepatomas, already described (section level 2, p. 96):
– Peripheral opacification of the tumors (26)
– Arteriovenous shunt with simultaneous opacification of the aorta (17) and the branches (10, 11) of the right branch of the portal vein

28

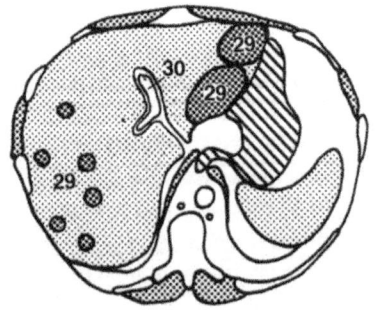

This image ends the series on hepatomas and serves at the same time as transition to the following series, that on metastases.

Note the multiple hypodensities (29) scattered all over the hepatic parenchyma.

This indicates either a diffuse hepatoma or multiple metastases. Only the clinical and biological data permit diagnosis. A puncture biopsy of the liver leads in this case to the diagnosis of diffuse hepatoma (section level 1, p. 95).
30 Branch of the portal vein

These two scans were taken in a 60-year-old woman examined due to changes in general condition.

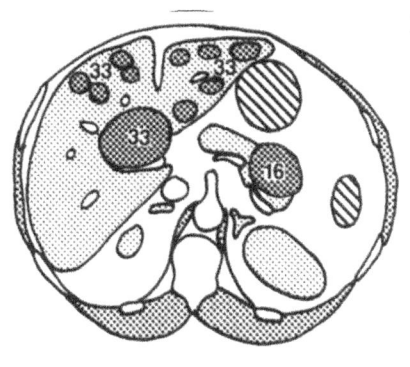

The multiplicity of lesions and their hypodense appearance (+20 HU), relatively well-delimited, suggest a secondary malignant involvement, although a diffuse hepatoma cannot be positively ruled out. **b** (section level 4, p. 98), however, confirms the hypothesis of a pancreatic carcinoma (*16*) with metastases in the liver (*33*).

These scans demonstrate the two common characteristics of metastases to the liver: multiplicity and hypodensity.

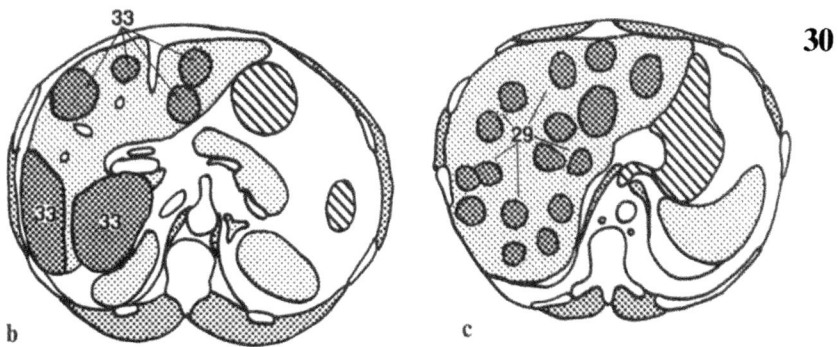

b   c

These four scans have been performed prior to and following contrast injection in two patients.

a and **b** (section level 4, p. 98) demonstrate the typical appearance of multiple liver metastases (*33*):

– Hypodense prior to contrast injection
– Discrete opacification following injection, clearly less important than that of the normal parenchyma, so that the differential density is increased (the metastases are better visible)

c and **d** (section level 1, p. 95) show a possibility which, although less frequent, must nevertheless be noted: the disappearance after contrast injection of metastases (*29*) which had previously been well visible. (The opposite case may also occur: metastases are seen only after contrast injection.) The search for liver metastases must therefore always be carried out both before and after contrast injection. This technical matter serves to remind us of the following fundamental points:

– There are visible hypodense metastases which accentuate their differential density since they poorly take up iodine whereas the normal parenchyma takes up much more
– There are invisible isodense metastases which appear after intravenous contrast injection because of the disharmonious uptake by parenchyma and tumor
– There are visible hypodense metastases which disappear after contrast injection because they accumulate enough contrast to become isodense

31
32
33

These images have in common that they illustrate less typical appearances of liver metastases.

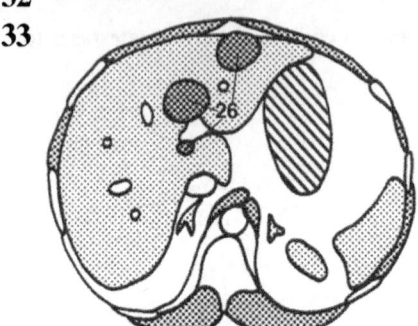

31a, b (section level 2, p. 96): Cystic metastases (*26*) of a malignant melanoma (before and after contrast injection). The wall is occasionally thicker, with irregular inner contours which are more evocative. Besides melanomas, ovarian, colic, and pulmonary tumors can also develop necrotic areas and cysts.

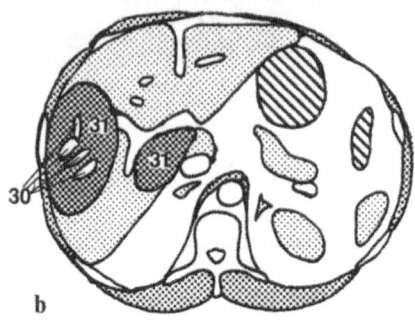

b

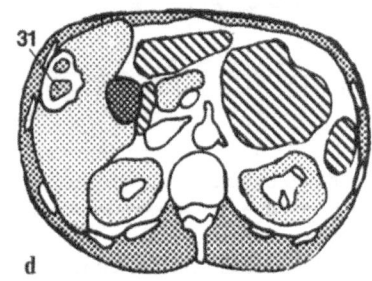

d

32a–d: Calcified metastases of an ovarian (**a, b**) and of a colic (**c, d**) neoplasm. **a** and **b** (section level 3, p. 97) are characteristic, with central calcifications (*30*) surrounded by a hypodense tumoral halo (*31*) which allows the differentiation of metastasis from calcified benign tumor.

c and **d** (section level 5, p. 99) are far less suggestive (*31*) and could be misinterpreted, for instance, as a calcified granuloma. The multiplicity of lesions and the context (colic carcinoma) justify the diagnosis, however. Calcifying metastases are generally secondary to colic and ovarian tumors but can also be found, albeit less frequently, in breast and renal tumors and in melanomas.

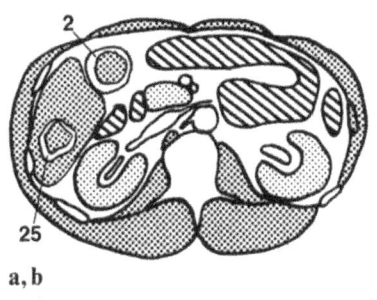
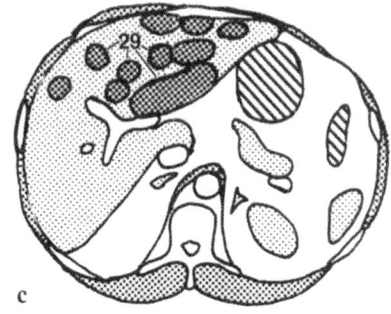

33a–c: Metastases in pathologic livers.

a, b (section level 6, p. 100): Metastasis (*25*) of a cancer of the sigmoid colon with a fatty liver. The mass is spontaneously dense before injection (scan 33a) and shows the typical ring-shaped enhancement after bolus injection (scan 33b). Note the thickened walls of the gallbladder (*2*).

c (section level 3, p. 97): Scan before contrast injection, showing a hemochromatosic, hyperdense liver. The entire left liver lobe and a part of the right liver are affected by metastases (*29*).

This scan is taken before contrast injection. **34**

Despite the absence of density measurements, one can conclude on the basis of two criteria that the liver, although homogeneous, has a density clearly below normal (the reader should refer here to section level 3, p. 97).

Hypodensity of the liver is indicated by:
- The hepatic and portal vessels appear denser than does the liver parenchyma, although no contrast has been injected.
- The density of the liver is clearly less marked than that of the spleen; normally the density of the liver is about 5–10 HU above that of the spleen.

Only one etiology suggests itself for this diffuse infiltration of the liver, namely steatosis.

Steatosis has multiple causes, among which the first is alcoholic cirrhosis; others include corticotherapy, hypercorticism, obesity, parenteral feeding, and diabetes.

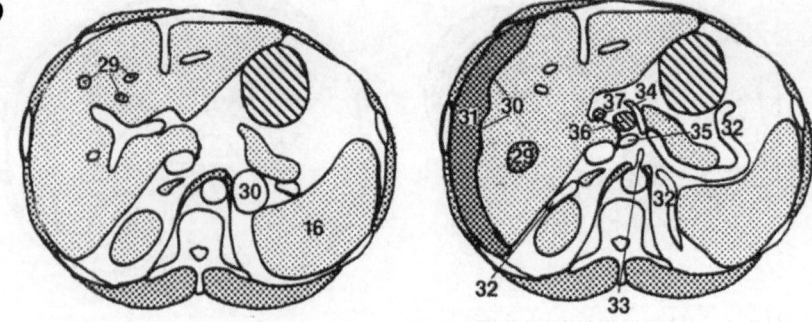

a (section level 2, p. 96): One recognizes here the perihepatic fluid effusion (*26*). But where is this exactly: sub- or extracapsular? Subcapsular, of course: this crescentlike appearance with obtuse connection angles to the parenchyma is typical of subcapsular effusion.

Most commonly this is a posttraumatic hematoma, sometimes following puncture biopsy or hepatectomy, but also concomitant with tumors. Nonhematic subcapsular liquid collections are rare.

b (section level 1, p. 95): In this case the diagnosis of hematoma (*29*) of the liver is more difficult:
- On the one hand, the typical crescent shape is not present
- On the other, its densities are low, since the hematoma is a long-standing one

Only the subcapsular location and, above all, the history of traumatism to the abdomen suggest this diagnosis rather than that of benign cyst.

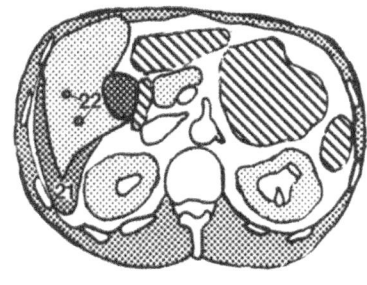

40

These two scans (**a, b**) were performed after contrast injection.

One notices here:
– Liver with discretely uneven contours (known cirrhosis) (section level 5, p. 99)
– Ascites localized around the liver (*21*)
– Dilatation of the intrahepatic bile ducts in the right liver lobe (*22*)

CT characteristics of intrahepatic bile duct dilatation are:
– Rounded or linear hypodensities
– Liquid-type density
– No enhancement following contrast injection
– A peculiar distribution, i. e., the hypodensities are always satellites to the portal vessels

These data rule out the two anomalies with which intrahepatic bile duct dilatation could be confused:
– Metastases: these have unknown distribution and are opacified after contrast injection
– Vascular dilatations: these are markedly opacified after contrast administration

The next step is to search for the etiology of this localized dilatation. If you have no idea here, examination of scan 41 is recommended.

This image provides the etiology of the localized dilatation of the intrahepatic **41** bile ducts of scan 40; it is a hematoma of the porta hepatis.

Let us use this example to review the etiology of such dilatations:
1. Tumor
   – primary hepatic (scans 26?, 40?, 41) or secondary
   – of the gallbladder
   – of the bile ducts
2. Infection
   – of the bile ducts
   – in alveolar echinococcosis (cf. scan 20)
3. Calculus
   – at the level of the porta hepatis
4. Traumatism (iatrogenic or not)

42

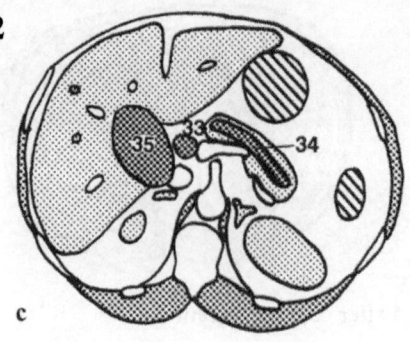

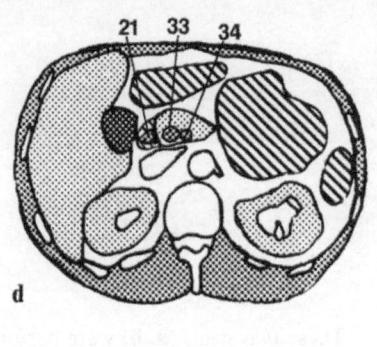

These four sections – porta hepatis (**a**), pedicular (**b**), pancreatic (**c**), and ampular (**d**) – were performed after contrast injection. **c** corresponds to section level 4 (p. 98), and **d**, to section level 5 (p. 99).

The fact that we have seen the dilatation of the intra- and extrahepatic bile ducts, Wirsung's canal, and gallbladder does not mean that we have *evaluated* this image: CT investigation, as any radiographic examination, aims at finding the cause of the dilatation.

Let us consider the characteristics of this image:
- Marked dilatation of the intra- and, especially, the extrahepatic bile ducts
- Very low situated obstacle, since the common bile duct (*33*) is dilated up to its termination, as is Wirsung's duct (*34*)
- Associated dilatation of the gallbladder (*35*)
- No stone in the lower extremity of the common bile duct
- Poor opacification of the second part of the duodenum (*21*) (presence of a mass?)

These findings strongly suggest a tumoral origin; in surgery a malignant tumor of the second part of the duodenum was, in fact, found.

Before ending this series let us review briefly the various etiologies of bile duct dilatations and their characteristics:

1. Tumor (pancreatic or biliary)
- very marked dilatation of the extra- and intrahepatic bile ducts
- sudden change in the caliber of the common bile duct, the lower extremity of which is often irregular
- visibility of the tumor
- often associated is dilatation of the gallbladder with vascular and retroperitoneal invasion

2. Pancreatitis
- minimal or moderate dilatation of the bile ducts
- fusiform progressive dilatation without sudden change in the caliber
- no dilatation of the gallbladder
- possible calcifications of chronic pancreatitis

3. Calculi
- moderate dilatation of the bile ducts
- fusiform caliber or sudden change in the caliber
- calculus visible in 80%–90% of cases

Is this also a dilatation of the intrahepatic bile ducts? No. (section level 2, p. 96)

The anomaly is located at the level of the bile ducts, as shown by the characteristic distribution; it is not liquid but air (26).

Several years earlier the patient had undergone choledocoduodenal anastomosis, which accounts for the presence of air in his bile ducts. Note also the presence of left pleural effusion.

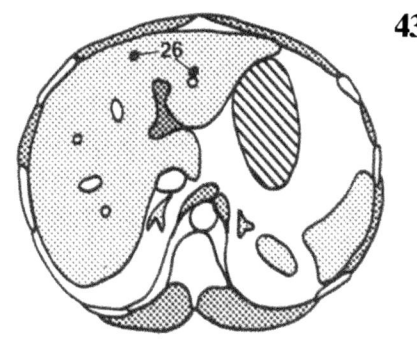

43

We might note here the other possible etiologies of aerobilia:
- Catheterization of the sphincter of Oddi
- Gallstone ileus
- Carcinoma of the bile ducts, duodenum, stomach, pancreas, or colon
- Ectopic orifice of the common bile duct (in the third or even fourth part of the duodenum)

While CT is not the best method for searching for gallstones (21), one must be able to recognize them, as on this scan (section level 5, p. 99).

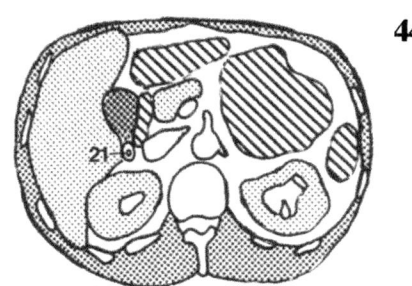

44

45

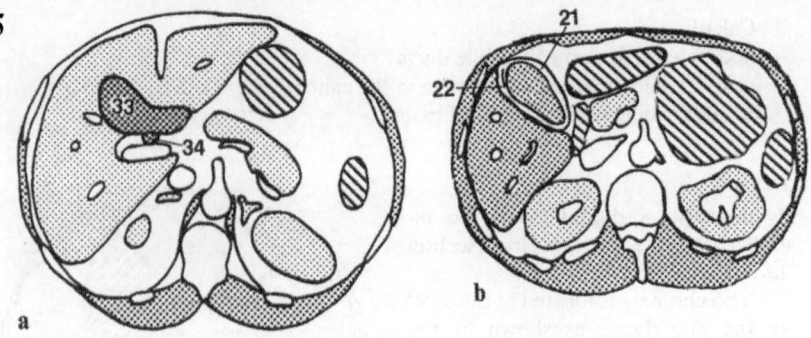

These two scans refer to two different patients. In **a** (section level 4, p. 98) one notices:
- Gallbladder (*33*) of increased volume, with a diameter above 5 cm
- Regular thickening of the entire gallbladder wall
- Contrast uptake by the gallbladder wall after contrast injection

These are the CT criteria of cholecystitis, often accompanied by the presence of fluid in the gallbladder bed (not in this case). Note the dilatation of the common bile duct (*34*) above a calculus.

b should remind one of scan 33. This patient with a liver metastasis in a fatty liver also has another disease: gangrenous cholecystitis or empyema. The three CT criteria which indicate this are (section level 5, p. 99):
- Thickening of the gallbladder wall with obvious contrast uptake after its administration (*21*)
- Air in the gallbladder wall (*22*)
- Gallbladder contents denser than "normal" bile

Let us consider these features in detail:
- The normal thickness of the gallbladder wall is always less than 2 mm; in cholecystitis it can reach 5–10 mm
- In gangrenous cholecystitis air can also be seen in the gallbladder proper
- Bile usually has a density of 0–20 HU (in scan **b** it has more than 30 HU)

This CT image provides more information about the above patient's way of life than would any questioning.

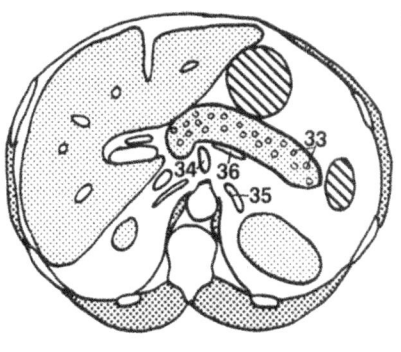

As should be clear, it concerns a patient with chronic alcoholism and a typical calcifying chronic pancreatitis (section level 4, p. 98). Parenchymatous calcifications (*33*) outline perfectly the entire pancreas, which here is almost horizontal, as is usual in shorter patients. The scan was taken just after bolus injection, so that the superior mesenteric artery (*34*) and the two renal arteries (*35*) are opacified, whereas the splenic vein (*36*), visible in the posterior concavity of the body of the pancreas, is not yet opacified. The liver parenchyma shows no CT sign of cirrhosis or of steatosis, despite the context.

Note the perfect renal corticomedullar differentiation obtained with the bolus injection.

This image is very characteristic (well-described), very specific (indicating a group of diseases), and even pathognomonic (permitting a precise diagnosis).

47

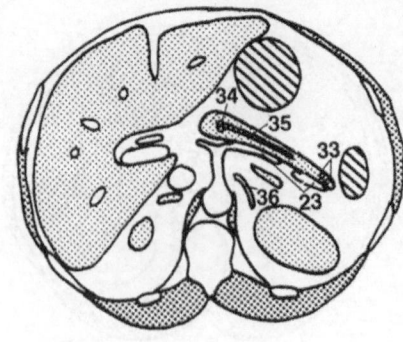

Several of the images here follow one another, but they do not all look alike, even in the same context.

This is also a chronic pancreatitis, but with only some calcifications in an atrophic pancreas with a dilated Wirsung's duct. This set of signs (section level 4, p. 98) is very specific and nearly pathognomonic. It is particularly useful because of the clearness of the sign, that is, because of the quality of the character, which renders it very "characteristic" (very typical):

- Pancreatic calcifications: intraparenchymatous (*33*) and/or intracanalicular (*34*)
- Decreased size of the pancreas
- Dilatation, often irregular or monoliform, of Wirsung's duct (*35*), and less frequently of the common bile duct

Note also the presence of intra-abdominal fat separating the various organs and thus permitting their correct visualization. The left renal vein (*36*) is already visible.

48

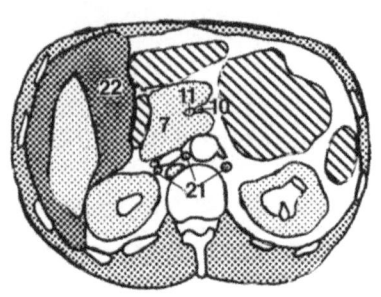

Observation of this image (section level 5, p. 99) yields the following points:

- The head of the pancreas is increased in volume, irregular, ill-delimited, and heterogeneous (*7*)
- The mesenteric vessels are hemmed within the pancreatic mass (*10, 11*)
- The fatty line which normally separates the pancreatic head from the vena cava (*9*) does not exist
- There are hypertrophic lumboaortic retroperitoneal ganglions (*21*)
- There are no pancreatic calcifications
- There is ascites present (*22*)

We may conclude from these observations a carcinoma of the head of the pancreas. It is an adenocarcinoma, the most frequent etiology of pancreatic tumors.

The presence of a further lesion in this patient will certainly have been noted, namely a solitary cyst in the right kidney. While this need not be included in the interpretation, it must be pointed out in the comment.

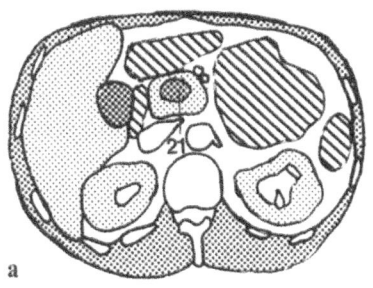 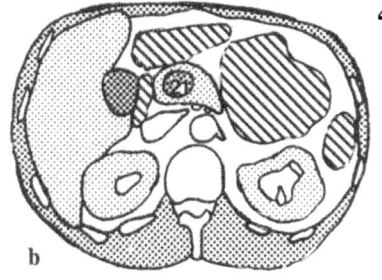

a   b

As we know, CT images alone, with certain exceptions, do not permit histologic diagnosis. They can only afford elements for orientation which may be combined with clinical and biological data.

There are two illustrations of this (section level 5, p. 99). These two scans (**a**, **b**) show the head of the pancreas; it is increased in volume, heterogeneous, with a central low-density zone (*21*). The superior mesenteric vessels and the inferior vena cava are separated from it by a fatty line. There are neither calcifications nor ganglions – negative signs which take on a great value for constructing one's reasoning. The first case (**a**) concerns a partially necrotic adenocarcinoma, the second (**b**) chronic pancreatitis with pseudocyst. These results lead us to discuss the various criteria for the diagnosis of adenocarcinoma of the pancreas.

This tumor results in:
Before contrast administration, deformation of the pancreas, mainly at the level of the head, the preferential site for this carcinoma; the mass is spontaneously iso- or hypodense.
After contrast administration, a hypodense mass, since the tumor is poorly vascularized and remains in contrast with the density of the normal pancreatic parenchyma which is enhanced, depending on the technique utilized.

Depending on its site, canalicular involvement must be sought: regular and often marked dilatation of Wirsung's duct, marked dilatation of the common bile duct with irregular appearance of its lower extremity, and retention cysts.

Extension to neighboring organs (stomach, spleen, colic angle) and to the vessels (mesenteric artery and vein, portal vein, celiac trunk, splenic vein) results in disappearance of the fatty line normally separating the pancreas from these various structures. Involvement of the lymph nodes begins with the superior mesenteric and the celiac nodes and extends later to the lumboaortic and interaorticocaval nodes.

Metastases to the liver are common, whereas ascites is rare.

50

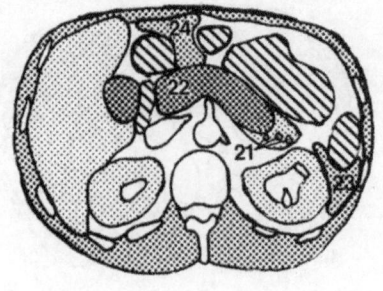

When ultrasonography of the abdomen showed in this patient with chronic pancreatitis a cystlike lesion in the head of the pancreas, CT investigations were requested (section level 5, p. 99).

CT scans demonstrate calcifications (21) in the tail of the pancreas as well as the presence of a hydric density (22) in the head of the pancreas, which was formerly referred to as a pseudocyst in calcifying chronic pancreatitis.

Surgery uncovered a primary colloid cancer of the pancreas with diffuse peritoneal metastases.

A second look at these scans will show a slightly dense and fixed appearance in the upper part of the left parietocolic recess (23) and the mesentery (24), anterior to the head of the pancreas. These anomalies should attract one's attention: they indicate the peritoneal dissemination.

51

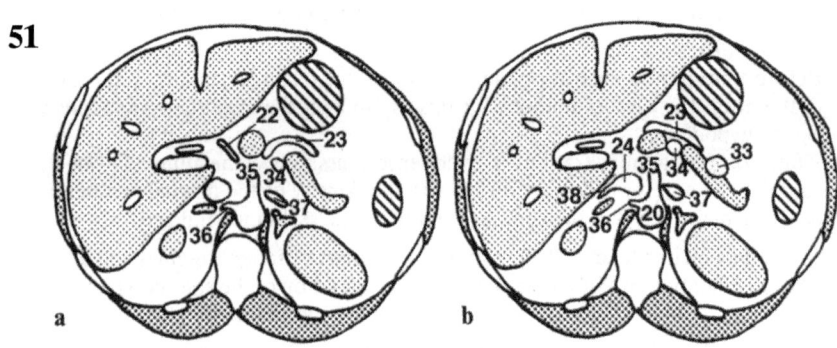

| 34 Splenic vein | 36 Right renal artery | 38 Right renal vein |
| 35 Superior mesenteric artery | 37 Left renal vein | |

Do these scans (section level 4, p. 98) show a normal image of the pancreas? No; the patient has an insulinoma (33) which at first was mistaken for a loop of the splenic artery (23).

The scans illustrate the difficult diagnosis of this small, hypervascularized tumor.

The search for an insulinoma requires a particular examination technique: two consecutive rapid sequences immediately after bolus injection. The request for such a procedure should be made clear with the support of clinical and biological data, specifying a "search for insulinoma."

The cysts **a** and **b** (*21*) in the head of the pancreas (section level 5, p. 99) have been demonstrated by echography, performed due to pain in the abdomen. **a** demonstrates a cystadenoma of the head of the pancreas. **b** shows a pseudocyst.

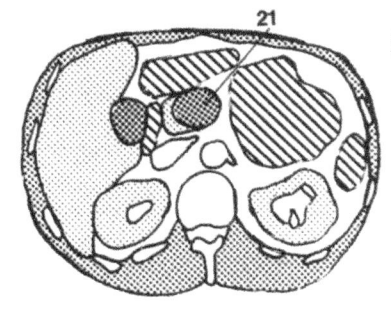

A lesion of the pancreas with liquid-type density may be any of the following:

- A pseudocyst (scans 49, 52b, 53, 54a, 56b)
- A necrotic tumor (scan 49), exceptionally a colloid tumor (scan 50)
- Congenital cysts in von Hippel-Lindau disease or in polycystic disease
- An infectious involvement – hydatid cyst, abscess (scan 56c)
- A primary cystic tumor – serous adenoma or cystadenoma (Table 1)

Table 1. Comparison of two primary cystic tumors

	Serous adenoma	Cystadenoma (**a**)
Size	< 2 cm	> 2 cm
Number of cysts	Numerous, small	< 10
Degeneration	Never	Precancerous stage degenerates into cystadenocarcinoma with appearance of a bud
Calcification	Frequent, central	Rare, septal
Localization	No preference	Rather in body or in tail

53

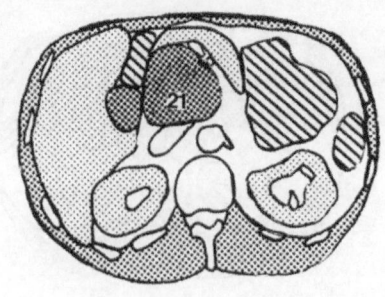

What is to be made of this image (section level 5, p. 99)?
1. The diagnosis of cyst (*21*) is obvious: rounded and well-delimited mass, with thin, smooth wall and liquid content.
2. Localizing the mass, however, is more difficult. Begin by locating the liver, gallbladder, and duodenum on the right, the inferior vena cava, aorta, and renal vessels behind; pancreas and mesenteric vessels are slightly more difficult to locate. Look more closely: these are displaced forwardly and laterally. Compare this image with that on p. 99, and you can easily conceptualize the displacements.
3. Interpretation of the two points of the comment is delicate:
   - for the origin of the mass is difficult to assess due to:
   - its important volume
   - the absence of any symptomatology – clinical, pancreatic, biliary, or digestive

It is, in fact, a pseudocyst of the pancreas.

54

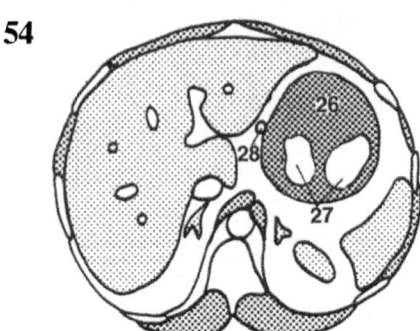

These scans permit us to analyze an identical image of two cases (**a** and **b**) (section level 2, p. 96):
On the right: liver and aorta
On the left: behind, the spleen; in front, a rounded and heterogeneous voluminous mass (*26*)
There are two types of hyperdensities: the one is diffuse and measures +80 HU (*27*), and the other has a metallic tonality (*28*).

One structure is missing: Does the mass correspond to the stomach?

a: No, the stomach is laminated anteriorly; its only visible part is that centered by the weighted gastric tube (*28*). The mass is a pancreatic pseudocyst with digestive fistula allowing the passage of Gastrografin (*27*).

b: Yes, the stomach is distended by recent digestive hemorrhage (*27*). Fresh blood is dense; the hyperdensity (*28*) is due to a metal clip, the patient having had gastrectomy 2–3 days previously.

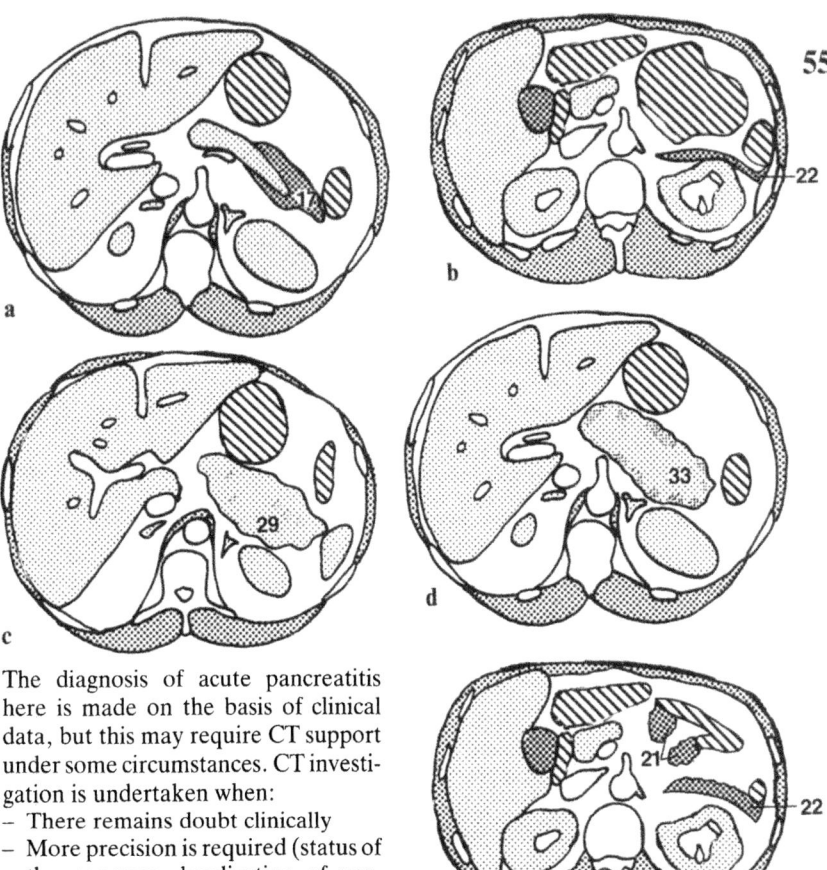

The diagnosis of acute pancreatitis here is made on the basis of clinical data, but this may require CT support under some circumstances. CT investigation is undertaken when:
– There remains doubt clinically
– More precision is required (status of the pancreas, localization of possible necrotic-hemorrhagic processes, and/or collections)

Scans 55a and b concern a patient with acute pancreatitis of the tail of the pancreas. **a** (section level 4, p. 98): Increased volume (*17*), heterogeneous appearance, and ill-defined contours in the tail of the pancreas. **b** (section level 5, p. 99): Thickening of the anterior pararenal fascia (*21*) and the left lateroconal fascia (*22*).

Scans 55c–e show acute pancreatitis of the body and tail of the pancreas; these present four further signs:
c (section level 3, p. 97), infiltration of the omental sac (*29*)
d (section level 4, p. 98), infiltration of the anterior pararenal space (*33*)
e (section level 5, p. 99), infiltration of the mesentery (*21*) and exudation penetrating into the left paracolic space (*22*).

A total of six signs are illustrated here, in order of decreasing frequency:
1. pancreatomegaly
2. thickening of the fasciae
3. left paracolic infiltration
4. infiltration of the omental sac
5. anterior pararenal infiltration
6. infiltration of the mesentery

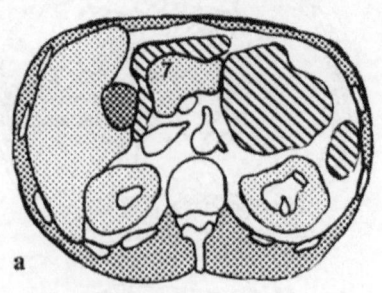 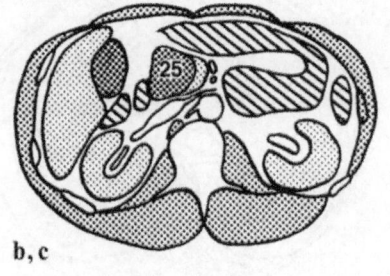

a   b, c

a, b (section level 5, p. 99) concern a case of acute pancreatitis of the head of the pancreas (7).

Note the markedly increased volume of the head with poorly defined limits and heterogeneous densities.

In the case of favorable development CT controls are performed after 3 and 6 weeks.

b (section level 6, p. 100) represents the control after 3 weeks and shows the head of the pancreas at the upper limit of normal volume and with clear contours. It still has a heterogeneous structure, with a rounded, hypodense, and well-delimited lesion (25). It is too early here to speak of a pseudocyst, since this hypodensity may yet resorb. Its persistence at the 6-week control would confirm the diagnosis of pseudocyst; it is usually thought that no changes occur after this time.

c (section level 6, p. 100) concerns another patient, who had undergone cephalic duodenopancreatectomy 3 weeks earlier and had been febrile for a few days. The rounded, hypodense lesion with walls taking up the contrast is an abscess of the pancreatic bed (25). The appearance may be less typical and may include a satellite mass possibly containing air. The presence of air suggests an abscess focus.

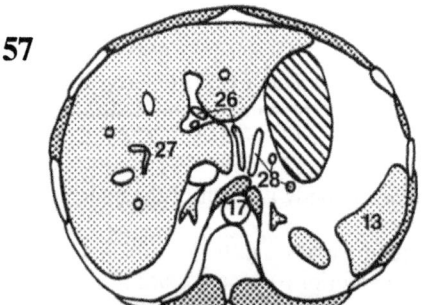

What can one make of the spleen (13) in this case (section level 2, p. 96)?

Scan **57a** was performed during bolus injection, as shown by the intense opacification of the aorta (17), the hepatic artery (26), its intraparenchymatous branches (27), and the splenic artery (28).

The initial, strongly heterogeneous and organized image of the splenic parenchyma is normal. This results from a peculiarity of the spleen, which has tissular compartments with variable blood flow.

Scan **b**: The splenic parenchyma (17) very quickly becomes homogeneous.

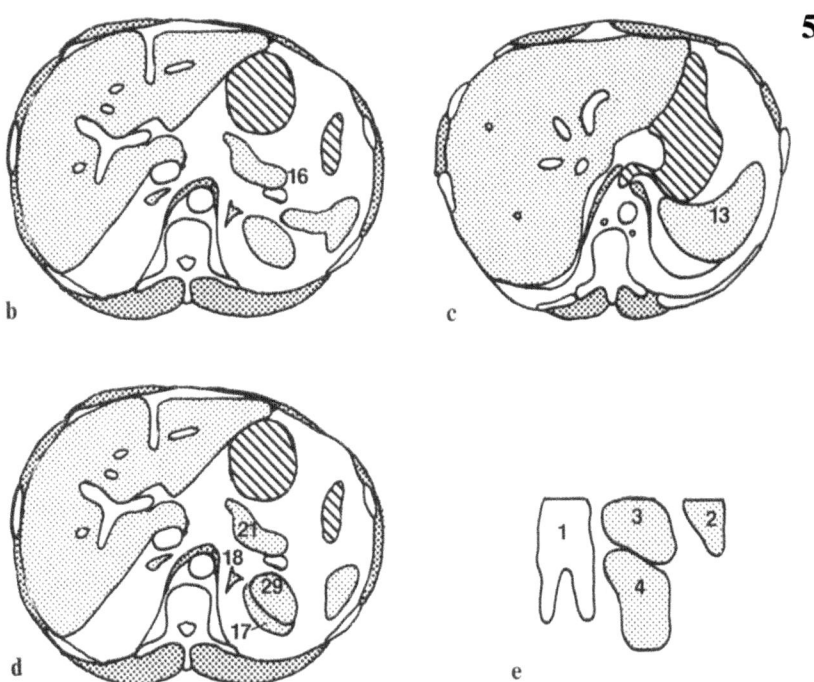

CT is only rarely utilized for examining the spleen. It is useful however to know the problems which may arise due to various conditions in this organ.

First example: **a** and **b** (section level 3, p. 97): This bilobate spleen (*16*) could be mistaken for a pancreatic (*21*), adrenal (*18*), or renal mass (*17*) in echography. The CT image demonstrates its splenic origin by showing, on the one hand, both its continuity with the splenic parenchyma and its simultaneous, similar opacification with that of the spleen, and, on the other, the integrity of the other organs.

Second example: **c, d, e**: Here is a supernumerary spleen. *Scan 58c* (section level 1, p. 95) demonstrates the spleen (*13*).
d (section level 3, p. 97) shows a mass in the right hypochondrium (*29*), distinct from the pancreas (*21*), the left adrenal (*18*), and the left kidney (*17*). It has the same density as the spleen.
e affirms the rupture in the continuity between the spleen (*1*) and the supernumerary spleen (*2*). Other notable parts include the spine (*3*) and left kidney (*4*).

59

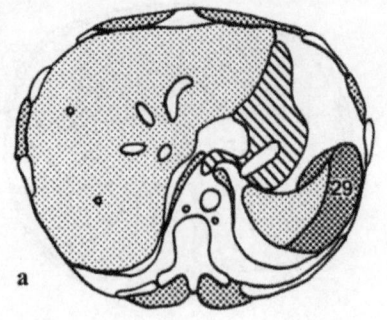 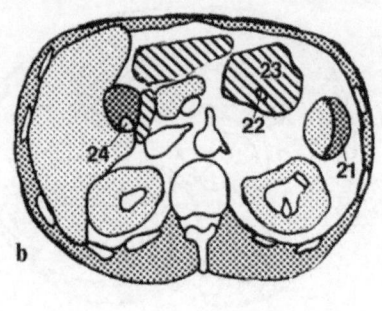

There is only one interpretation for these scans: long-standing subcapsular hematoma:

1. The lesion is peripheral, has a crescentlike appearance, and raises the capsule: it is therefore subcapsular
2. Its density is low, homogeneous, and unchanged after contrast injection: it is therefore liquid
3. Subcapsular liquid effusion of the spleen has only one etiology, i.e., old hematoma; although fresh blood has a high density, this can fall within the range of water during evolution of the hematoma

a (section level 1, p. 95) demonstrates, besides the hematoma of the spleen (*29*), a linear hyperdensity (*30*) in the stomach which corresponds to a stomach tube for aspiration.

b (section level 5, p. 99) also shows the hematoma (*21*), the stomach tube (*22*) in the stomach (*23*), as well as gallstones (*24*).

60

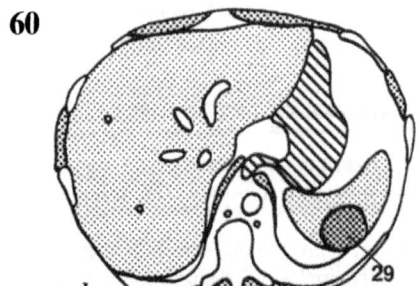 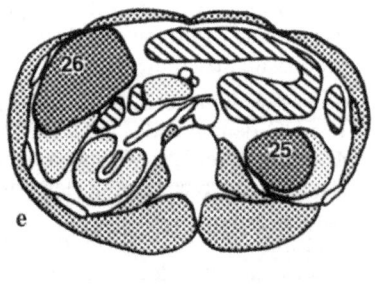

Splenic cysts are not uncommon. As elsewhere, these appear as rounded, well-delimited lesions, with fluid content, not enhanced by contrast injection. In some cases one finds contrast uptake in the cyst wall. The latter may also be calcified.

The two most frequent etiologies of splenic cysts are illustrated in scans 60a, b; others are presented in images 60c–e.

a (section level 1, p. 95): Splenic hematoma (*29*), posttraumatic. It may calcify.
b (section level 1, p. 95): Epithelial cyst (*29*).
c (section level 1, p. 95): Splenic infarct (*29*). In its initial phase this appears as a peripheral hypodense lesion, triangular, with lateral base. It may develop into a cyst, as in the case depicted here, or cicatrize and produce a notch at the periphery of the spleen.
d (section level 1, p. 95): A hydatid cyst (*29*).
e (section level 6, p. 100): The downward prolongation (*25*) and a hepatic localization (*26*) of the cyst in image 60d.

61

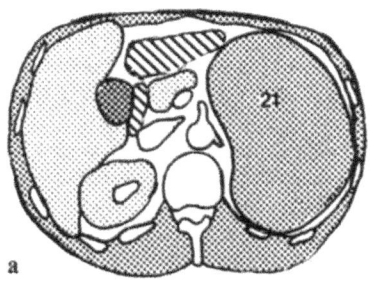

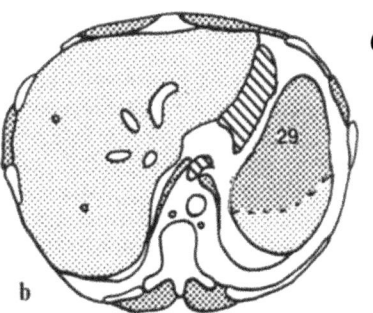

One will certainly have recognized enlargement of the spleen in both of these scans a and b and pointed out the heterogeneity of the structure. But now one must try to go further in the interpretation.

Apart from abscesses, heterogeneous spleen enlargements are related either to a lymphoma or to metastases.

a (section level 5, p. 99) depicts a lymphoma. Involvement of the spleen is seen as nodular, heterogeneous enlargement (*21*), but diagnosis requires the support of more elaborate data – that of imaging (adenopathies) as well as that of a clinical and a biological nature.

b (section level 1, p. 95) presents metastases (*29*). There often exists concomitant involvement of the liver (not in the case shown here). The causative primary cancer is variable. In this case it was an ovarian carcinoma – a frequent etiology, as are malignant melanoma and carcinoma of the lung and breast. The image indicates the criteria of metastases (hypodensity, multiplicity, polymorphism).

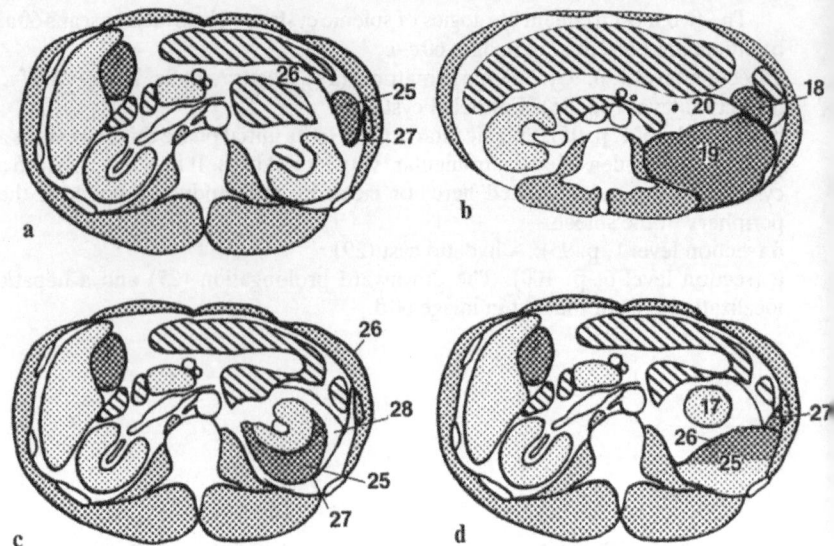

These four scans pass through the middle part of the abdomen. They have in common that the afflictions presented are located in the retroperitoneal space, although in different compartments.

a (section level 6, p. 100) demonstrates an appearance with which we are now familiar (see scan 55 e). We recognize the exudate in acute pancreatitis (25), with thickening of the anterior renal (26) and lateroconal (27) fasciae. The pancreas, the duodenum (except for the first segment), and the right and left colic angles belong to the anterior pararenal space, limited anteriorly by the posterior parietal peritoneum, behind by the anterior renal fascia, and laterally by the lateroconal fascia. The left and the right anterior pararenal spaces communicate on the median line. They also communicate on their inferior part, on the one hand, with the pelvis (as do all retroperitoneal spaces), and on the other, with the posterior pararenal space – which explains the presence of anomalies of the latter in pancreatitis.

b (section level 7, p. 101) is performed 2 cm below the previous slice and shows both the pancreatic exudate in the anterior pararenal space (18) and the involvement of the posterior pararenal space (19); the perirenal space (20), containing only the left ureter, is intact.

c (section level 6, p. 100) shows a perirenal hematoma (25). The perirenal space is limited anteriorly by the anterior renal fascia (26) and posteriorly by the posterior fascia (27). This space contains the kidney, the ureter, the adrenal gland, and perirenal fat separating the kidney from its fasciae. Here the anterior perirenal fat is visible (28), but behind, it is replaced by the hematoma (25), which comes into contact with the thickened posterior fascia (27).

d (section level 6, p. 100) shows the posterior pararenal space. When it is normal, as here on the right, it is virtual, situated between the posterior renal fascia and the fascia transversalis, and contains only lymph vessels and fat. On the left, a posterior pararenal hematoma comprising a horizontal sedimentation level (25) distends this space, displaces the kidney (17) forwardly, and thickens the posterior renal fascia (26) and the lateroconal fascia (27).

This brief review of the retroperitoneal space is justified by the necessity of indicating to the surgeon the precise location of the masses, abscesses, and hematomas of this region.

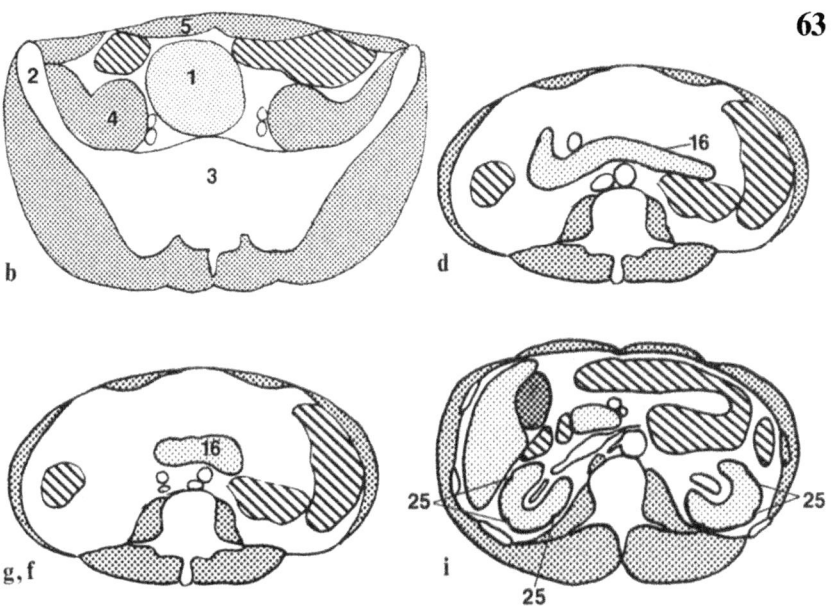

63

These images permit us to review our knowledge concerning congenital anomalies of the kidneys. These variants are known already since they also raise problems in conventional radiography and ultrasonography.

a, b: What should we think of this pelvic mass (*1*)? The answer is provided by scan **b** after contrast injection: pelvic kidney (*1*), upper part of the ilium (*2*), sacrum (*3*), iliopsoas muscle (*4*), rectus abdominis muscle (*5*), and iliac vessels (*6*).

c, d show another congenital anomaly: the horseshoe kidney (*16*), well displayed in 63d – which corresponds to section level 8, p. 101.

The four images **e–h**, performed at successive levels in the same patient show a sigmoid kidney (*16*). Slice **f** (section level 8, p. 101) is particularly demonstrative.

i (section level 6, p. 100) shows a normal anatomic variant: persistence in the adult of fetal lobulations (*25*).

64

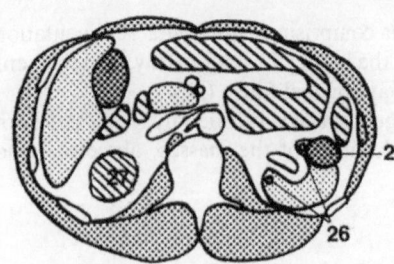

There should be no difficulty in preparing the comment and interpretation of this scan, corresponding to section level 6, p. 100: benign cyst of the left kidney (25).

The set of readable signs permits us to observe the following elementary points:
– Mass with fluid density
– Rounded
– Without walls
– Unchanged after contrast injection
– Absence of septations
– Clearly demarcated from the remaining parenchyma
– Absence of invasion of the sinusal adipose tissue and vessels

Note that besides the large cyst (25), with a diameter of 2 cm, there are two others of less than 5 mm (26).

What can we make of the right renal bed?
It is occupied by a part of the colon (27); this raises the possibility of ectopic kidney, agenesis of the kidney, or nephrectomy.

In the case presented, it is a result of nephrectomy, carried out 12 years earlier for adenocarcinoma.

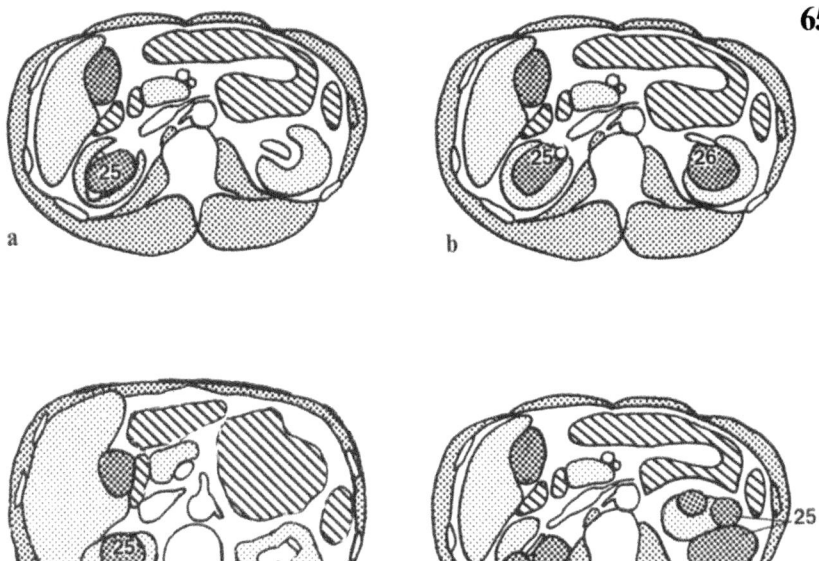

This series of four cysts (**a–d**) entails various problems for interpretation. The comment for these images, however, is easy.

a (section level 6, p. 100) shows a peculiar localization: a right parapyelic cyst (*25*) causing displacement of the pyelocaliceal cavities and the sinusal fat without invading them.

b (section level 6, p. 100): There is undisputably a parapyelic or sinusal cyst on the left (*25*) – but not the right, for this is a sinusal fibrolipomatosis (*26*) with fat densities of −50 HU.

c (section level 6, p. 100): The left renal parenchymatous hypodensity (*25*) could correspond to a benign cyst, but its density is elevated (+30 HU), and there is an irregular and ill-defined peripheral contrast uptake. In this 40-year-old woman, who had been subfebrile for 2 months with left lumbar pain, surgery discovered a cloudy fluid corresponding to a superinfected cyst. Infection is one of the causes of increased density of a benign cyst – in addition to hemorrhage, contamination by contrast material, calcifications, and artifacts due to a possible partial-volume effect.

d (section level 6, p. 100): The number of cysts (*25*) could suggest a polycystic disease. But here the context must be taken into account: the accidental finding of these cysts in a 60-year-old man, with no hypertension, with normal renal function, and without familial history of renal polycystosis, leads to the conclusion of multiple benign cysts.

66

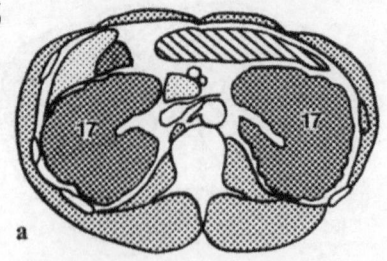
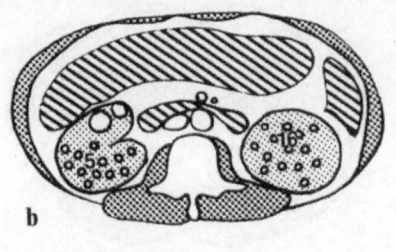

Both comment and interpretation regarding these two scans are easy.

a (section level 6, p. 100): Numerous cysts of variable size replace the renal parenchyma (*17*) which is now almost nonexistent and laminated between the cysts. This is the appearance of polycystic disease in the adult.

b (section level 7, p. 101): While roughly keeping their shape, the kidneys (*5, 16*) are quite voluminous (presence of multiple cysts of a size usually under 10 mm). This is the infantile form of polycystic disease.

67

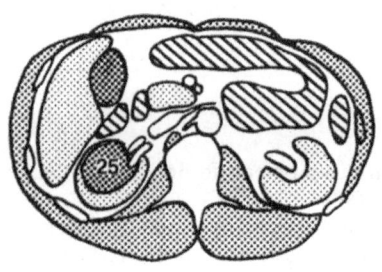

This image corresponds to section level 6 (see p. 100).

One notices here the anomaly in the right kidney. The anterior margin and the sinus of the kidney are occupied by a solid mass (*25*) which is less dense than the remaining parenchyma and has irregular contours. These signs suggest a malignant tumor, especially since the investigation has been performed due to hematuria and right lumbar pain.

It is an adenocarcinoma, by far the most frequent malignant renal tumor.
The CT characteristics are the following:
– Solid tumor
– More or less well-defined limits
– Hypodense with regard to the normal parenchyma after contrast injection, even heterogeneous, with a central area which does not take up the contrast (necrotic zone)
– At least partial obliteration of the sinusal fat with occasional invasion of the pyelocaliceal cavities
In such a case as this we need to search for:
   Extension beyond the capsule to the pararenal fascia and the adjoining organs
   Invasion of the vessels (renal vein, inferior vena cava)
   Lymph node involvement and metastases

The presence of these signs indicates malignancy and permits classification into one of four stages:

Stage I   tumor does not extend beyond the renal capsule
Stage II tumor extends beyond the capsule but remains within the fasciae
Stage III tumor invades the renal vein or the lymph nodes
Stage IV tumor invades other organs (proximity or metastases)

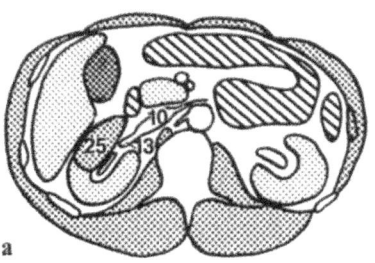 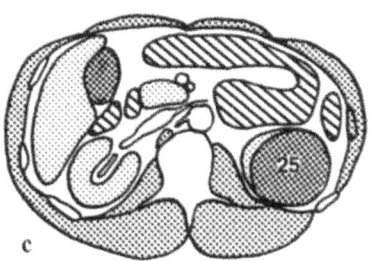

These two cases of renal adenocarcinoma have a common point despite their evident differences: they are both of stage I, i.e., the tumor does not extend beyond the renal capsule.

a and **b** (section level 6, p. 100): A well-delimited tumor (*25*) which displaces without invading the sinusal fat. The renal vein (*13*) and the inferior vena cava (*10*) are perfectly permeable and not deformed.

c and **d** (section level 6, p. 100): Observing the inferior vena cava (*10*) on scan **c**, one might think – although incorrectly – that this is either a thrombus or an invasion. However, it is simply a delayed opacification of the inferior vena cava with regard to the renal veins during bolus injection. Scan **d**, taken shortly thereafter, confirms the integrity of the inferior vena cava. There is thus also a stage I development of an adenocarcinoma (*25*).

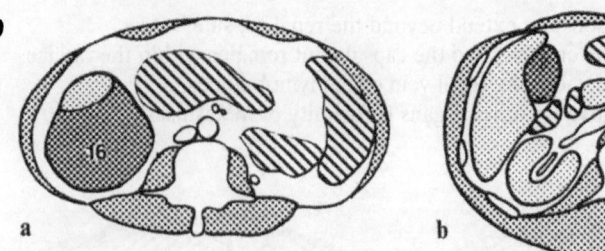

In terms of the classification into four stages as elaborated in scan 67, we easily recognize stage II, characterized by rupture of the capsule by a tumor that remains within the pararenal fasciae (69a), or stage III of the here more advanced tumor (69b).

a (section level 8, p. 101): A tumor with posteroinferior polar development (*16*) which has invaded the posterior perirenal fat but remains within the posterior pararenal fascia. Surgery confirmed the integrity of this fascia and of the psoas muscle.

b (section level 6, p. 100): Stage III, as characterized by invasion of the renal vein and/or presence of lymph node involvement (*25*). This image is a perfect illustration of stage III.

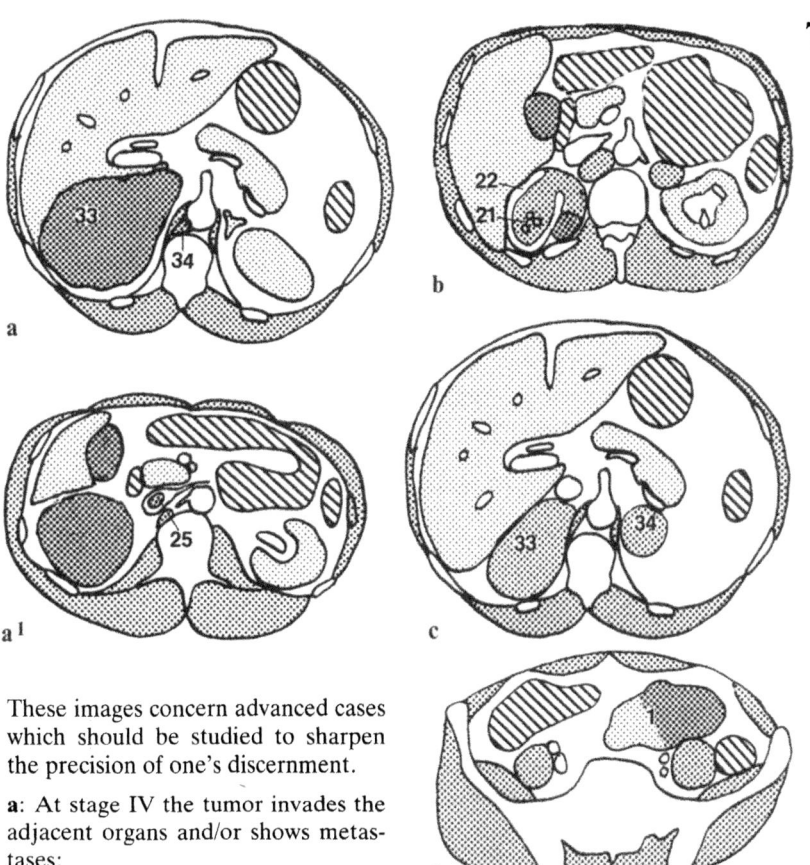

These images concern advanced cases which should be studied to sharpen the precision of one's discernment.

a: At stage IV the tumor invades the adjacent organs and/or shows metastases:

- Above (section level 4, p. 98), carcinoma invading by contiguity the posterior part of the right liver (*33*); there is right retrocrural lymph node enlargement (*34*) behind the crus of the diaphragm
- Below, on the left (section level 6, p. 100), the inferior vena cava is obliterated by an intraluminal thrombus and/or tumoral invasion (*25*)
- Below, on the right, the vein is again permeable

b, c: Another example of stage IV, with calcified right renal adenocarcinoma with metastases in both suprarenal glands. **b** (section level 5, p. 99). The right (*23*) and left (*26*) suprarenal metastases are even more clearly visible than in **c**. Note the two types of tumoral calcification:

- The more frequent central intratumoral calcifications (*21*)
- Much less frequent peripheral calcifications (*22*) similar to those seen in benign renal cysts

d: Observe the pelvic mass (*1*): this is a necrotic and calcified carcinoma in a left pelvic kidney.

71

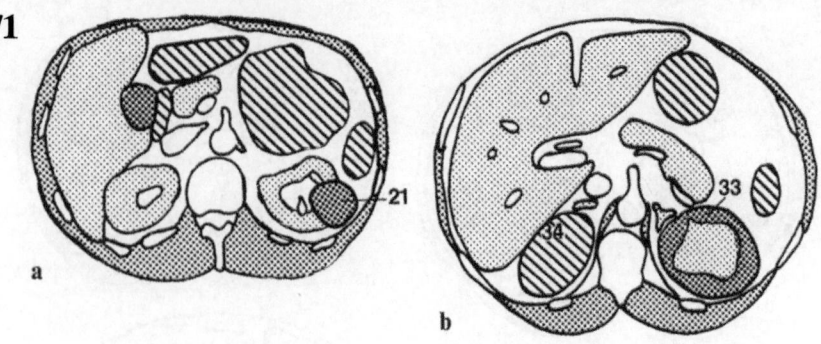

These two images (**a** and **b**) illustrate the appearance which a benign renal tumor may take on with three tissular components (adipose, muscular, and vascular).

a (section level 5, p. 99): The angiomyolipoma (*21*) is a solid tumor with a density after contrast injection from −150 HU (fat) to +150 HU (muscles and mainly the vessels, which are well opacified), well-delimited, but not encapsulated. Its diameter (in the present case 2.5 cm) is usually over 2 cm. This uncommon tumor occurs most frequently in subjects without particular antecedents.

b (section level 4, p. 98): It is useful to know the particular circumstance that the great majority of patients with tuberous sclerosis (Bourneville's disease) have an angiomyolipoma (*33*). **b** shows such an example; note the occupation of the right renal bed by colon (*34*) following nephrectomy. This pathology is useful to know, since the CT appearance is generally sufficient for diagnosis and can thus avoid further investigations (and intervention). The greatest prudence is recommended, however, since atypical appearances can be due to a liposarcoma.

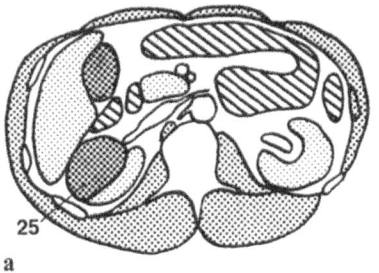

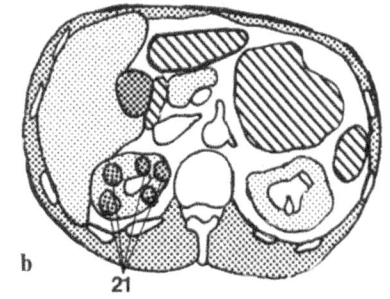

We are confronted here with severe interpretation problems. While it is certainly not difficult to write a comment on these masses, remember that besides the adenocarcinoma – albeit by far the most frequent malignant tumor of the kidney – there are other malignant involvements. These are illustrated by the three images (a–c) presented here.

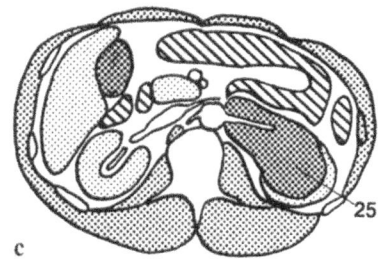

a (section level 6, p. 100) shows the infiltration of the right kidney by an irregular mass which is hypodense after contrast injection and consistent with a lymphoma (25). Further signs of lymphomas include diffuse increase of the renal volume without identifiable mass and the presence of multiple hypodense nodules either causing or not causing increase in the size of the kidney.

b (section level 5, p. 99) concerns multiple metastases (21) from a lung carcinoma. When there is a unique metastasis, this often cannot be differentiated from the primary tumor. Breast, stomach, colon, and pancreas can also metastasize to the kidney. The renal tumor then reveals the primary tumor, namely pancreatic carcinoma.

c (section level 6, p. 100): CT data does not permit the histologic diagnosis of this liposarcoma (25), but it allows assessment of its extension. This was surgically verified: involvement of the aorta (9) and of the left renal artery (26), as well as (on a higher-located slice not shown here) adherence to the stomach and spleen.

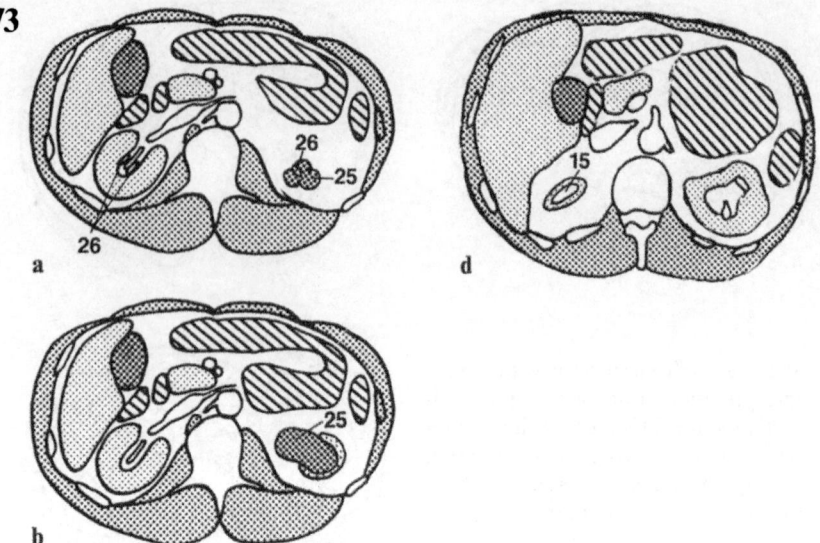

We have now come to the problem of small kidneys. These are usually unilateral and are accidental findings. They raise three possibilities: pyelonephritis, obstacle, and hypoplasia.

a (section level 6, p. 100): The small kidney in chronic pyelonephritis is easily recognized by its irregular, uneven contours (*25*), due to scars extending from the renal pelvis to the cortex, and due to the absence of pyelocaliceal dilatation. Calcification of the parenchyma can be found in the scarred areas. Note the lithiasis on the right and on the left (*26*) of the scan (before contrast injection).

b–d: In some cases the small kidney has smooth contours with pyelocaliceal dilatation (*25*). This is seen in obstructive uropathy (**b**) (section level 6, p. 100). When there is no dilatation, it is a matter of hypoplasia (**d**) (section level 5, p. 99).

c demonstrates the cause of the hydronephrosis seen in **b**: advanced carcinoma of the prostate.

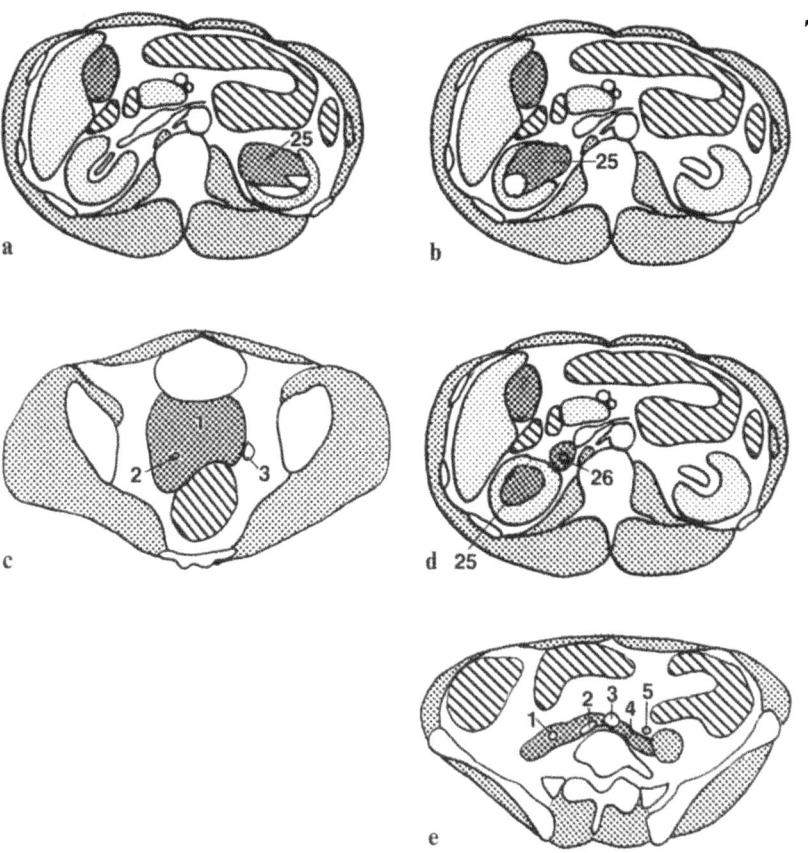

Dilatation of the pyelocaliceal cavities can be readily identified here. It is, however, necessary to go beyond this comment and interpret the observation.

a (section level 6, p. 100) demonstrates marked pyelocaliceal dilatation (*25*) with a double liquid/liquid level between the opaque and the nonopaque urine. A subjacent slice (not shown here) showed a stop on a stone which had been radiolucent at intravenous urography.

b, c (section level 6, p. 100) show right hydronephrosis (*25*). The carcinoma of the uterus (*1*) enclosing the right ureter (*2*) is responsible for the hydronephrosis, whereas the left ureter (*3*) is still patent (**c**).

d (section level 6, p. 100) shows right ureterohydronephrosis (*25*) related to retroperitoneal fibrosis (**e**). The opacity within the ureter corresponds to a derivation catheter (*26*).

e depicts the right ureter (*1*), inferior vena cava (*2*), and aorta (*3*) enclosed by fibrous tissue (*4*). The left ureter (*5*) is still permeable anterior to the retroperitoneal fibrosis (*4*).

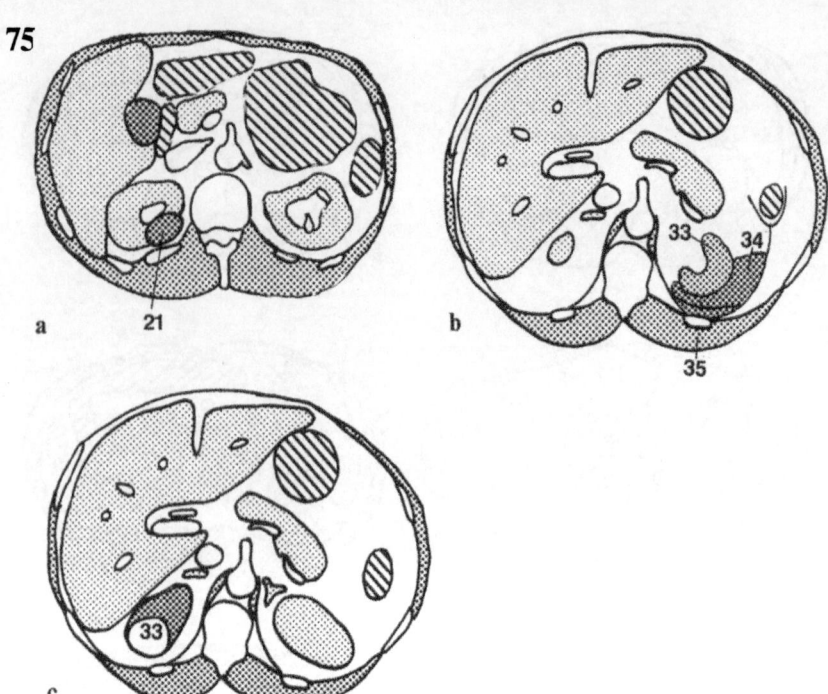

a

21

b

33 34

35

c

33

The common factor in this set of images is infection.

a (section level 5, p. 99): The hypodense and heterogeneous zone (*21*) in the middle part of the right kidney is an abscess secondary to ascending, retrocecal, suppurative appendicitis.

b (section level 4, p. 98): This is another renal abscess (*33*) with extension to the perirenal area (*34*), the posterior pararenal space, and the posterior muscles (*35*). Note the presence of air, a reliable sign of an abscess.

c (section level 4, p. 98): This scan, performed before contrast injection, shows a solid, rounded, totally calcified mass (*33*) in the upper pole of the right kidney. There was no change after contrast injection. Various etiologies must be considered:

– Calcification of a long-standing hematoma
– Totally calcified tumor
– Infection (tuberculosis, hydatidosis, etc.)

In fact, it is a case of calcifying renal tuberculosis.

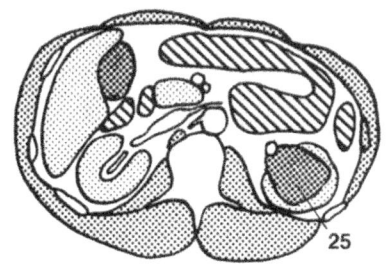

This complicated image concerns a case of hematuria (section level 6, p. 100) in a patient undergoing anticoagulative treatment. Should we consider the hematuria as only symptomatic or as revealing a subjacent lesion?

The CT image performed 2 days after the hematuric episode shows an abnormal left renal sinus with the following characteristics:
– Presence of a hypodense and heterogeneous mass (*25*) in the renal sinus
– Consequent disappearance of the sinusal fat
– Consequent poor filling of the renal pelvis

Etiologies to be discussed in this case are the following:
– Tumor of the excretory passages
– Clot
– Stone

The patient refused surgery, but a control investigation showed normal data. The image was thus very likely that of a clot.

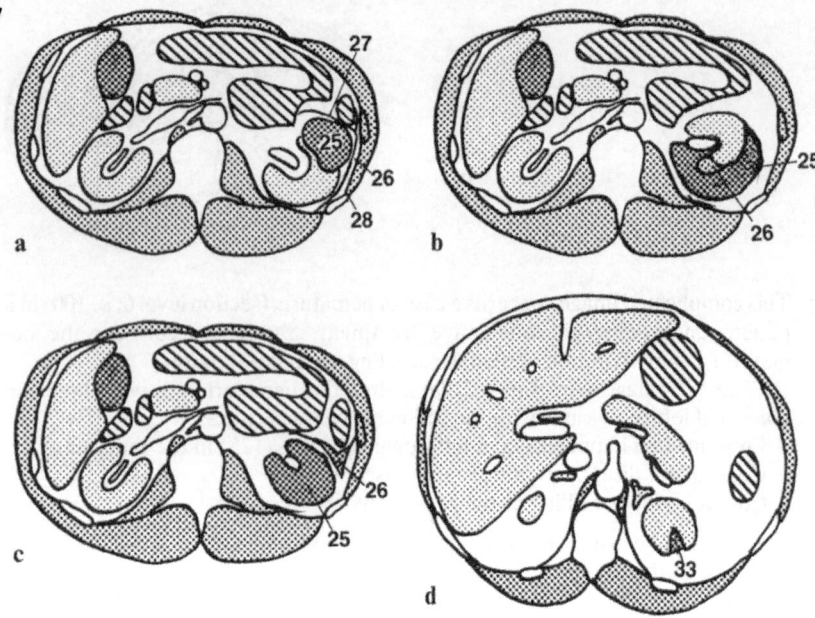

a (section level 6, p. 100): The etiology of this subcapsular hematoma (*25*) of the left kidney could be:
- Traumatic
- Tumoral
- Iatrogenic

In this case there is a double origin: a small adenocarcinoma of the left kidney is revealed by a hematoma in a patient with anticoagulative treatment.

Note that the perirenal space (*26*) is free and that the anterior (*27*) and posterior (*28*) fasciae are clearly visible.

b, c: What are the renal lesions in these two patients with traumatism to the abdomen?

b (section level 6, p. 100): A perirenal hematoma (*25*) should always lead to the search for a renal lesion. In this case there is an incomplete laceration (*26*), as there is no contrast-material extravasation.

c (section level 6, p. 100): The almost complete lack of opacification of the renal parenchyma (*25*) is the sign of incomplete laceration. There is, however, no associated hematoma, as in scan 77b. The presence of fluid (*26*) in the greater peritoneal cavity is due to puncture dialysis.

d (section level 6, p. 100): The triangular-shaped hypodensity with cortical base (*33*) suggests an ischemic process. This is the result of trauma.

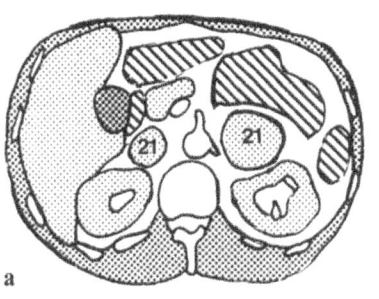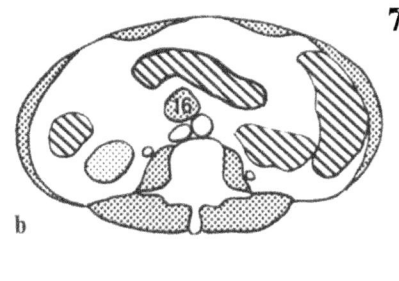

On **a** (section level 5, p. 99) one recognizes two voluminous, heterogeneous masses (*21*) anterior to the upper pole of the kidneys.

The question then arises as to whether these masses are independent or do they belong to an abdominal organ? On the right, they are clearly distinct from the duodenum (*3*), pancreas (*7*), inferior vena cava (*9*), and right kidney (*15*) and, on the left, from the loops of the small intestine (*4*), spleen (*22*), and left kidney (*15*). They are situated anterior to the upper pole of both kidneys. The masses thus correspond to pathological adrenal glands.

The possible etiologies of voluminous, bilateral suprarenal masses are:
1. pheochromocytoma
2. metastases

Clinical and biological data settle the question here. The symptomatology of pheochromocytomas is characterized particularly by bouts of hypertension and increased rates of catecholamines and their urinary derivates. In 90% of cases the pheochromocytoma is suprarenal, but it should be kept in mind that there do exist ectopic forms along the spine, for example, the abdominal (*16*) form in **b** (section level 8, p. 101), as well as the pelvic and intrathoracic forms.

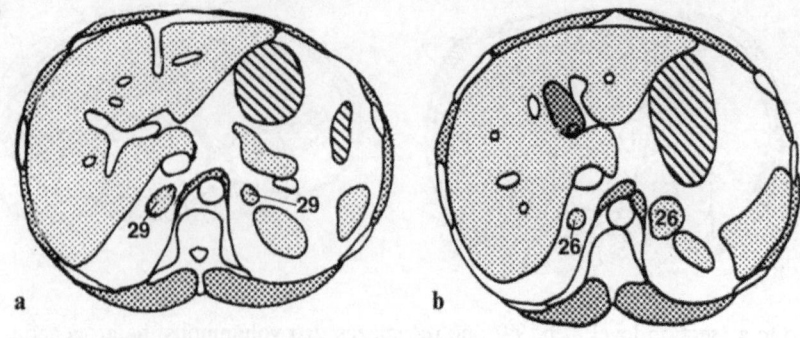

The possible etiologies in this case – with bilaterally increased volume of the suprarenal glands (cf. scan 78) – are:
1. Pheochromocytoma (scan 78)
2. Metastases (**b**)
3. Bilateral suprarenal hematoma (**a**) – much less frequently

a (section level 3, p. 97): The third of these possible etiologies is rare, especially in the adult, and, when bilateral as here, is accompanied by acute adrenal insufficiency. The hematoma (*29*) is recent, since the adrenals have a density of +60 to +80 HU, corresponding to that of fresh blood.

b (section level 2, p. 96): Unlike the two other etiologies, suprarenal metastases (*26*) are only exceptionally accompanied by an endocrine symptomatology. The following points favor this etiology:
– Bilaterality
– Large size
– Frequent necrosis
– Irregular contours
– Calcifications (rare)

These arguments merely suggest the diagnosis; only puncture biopsy would confirm it. Note also that this patient has gallbladder lithiasis (*27*).

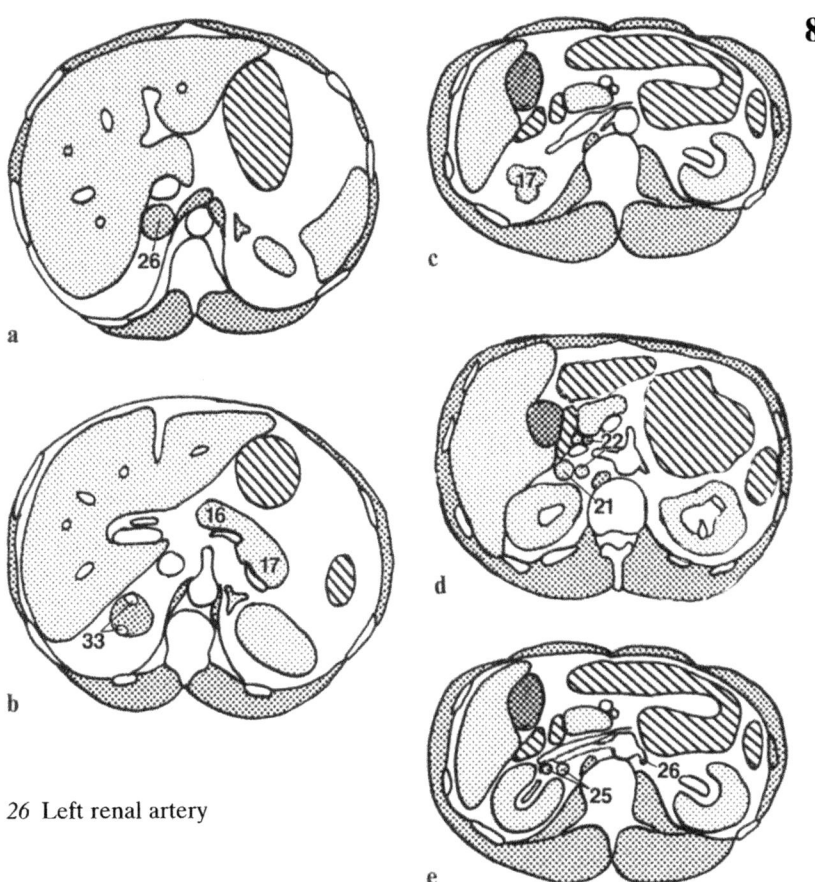

26 Left renal artery

These two cases allow us to discuss the problems raised by tuberculosis.

a–c: Nonevolutive, long-standing renal and suprarenal tuberculosis. These scans **a–c** are of a 70-year-old woman with high blood pressure, in whom urography revealed a *mute right kidney*. **a** (section level 2, p. 96): The hypodense lesion (*26*) with a diameter of 5 cm is a cyst with caseiform contents. **b** (section level 4, p. 98): Calcifications (*33*). Note also the lipomatous involution of the pancreas (*16, 17*). **c** (section level 6, p. 100): Uneven and cystic small right kidney (*17*).

d, e: Evolutive tuberculosis of the suprarenal gland. These scans are from a 35-year-old man of north African origin, presenting with right subcostal pain without particular antecedents. **d** (section level 5, p. 99): The right suprarenal gland (*21*) is increased in volume with a central hypodensity. There are several lymph node enlargements (*22*) around the large vessels. **e** (section level 6, p. 100): This scan, performed after bolus injection, permits differentiation between vessels and lymph node enlargements (*25*).

81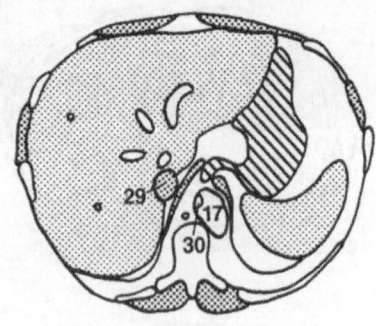

One notices in this scan, taken after contrast injection (section level 1, p. 95), a large right suprarenal gland (*29*).

As possible diagnoses in this patient without known endocrine pathology one would consider: adenoma, nonfunctional carcinoma, or metastasis.

Table 2 summarizes the CT characteristics of these various diagnostic hypotheses.

Table 2. The CT characteristics of adenoma, carcinoma, and metastases

	Adenoma	Carcinoma	Metastases
Localization	Unilateral	Unilateral	Bilateral
Size	Inf. to 3 cm	Sup. to 3 cm	Variable
Calcification	Rare	Frequent	Rare
Density	Low	Heterogeneous, since necrosis is frequent	Heterogeneous, when the size is above 2 cm as necrosis is then frequent
Contours	Regular	Irregular	Irregular
Miscellaneous	Absence of evolution	Hepatic and pulmonary metastases; invasion by contiguity	Primary carcinoma: lungs, kidney, thyroid, skin (melanoma), colon

These parameters are not definitive. Only puncture biopsy allows confirmation of the diagnosis.

The appearance here is quite suggestive of nonfunctional adenoma; this was confirmed only by absence of evolution after a 5-month interval.

In observing the aorta of this 70-year-old patient one notices:
– The walls are calcified (*30*), which is a sign of the presence of an atheroma
– The transverse diameter is increased, which could suggest an aneurysm.

However, the aorta has an ovoid appearance, and overlying and underlying slices show that this is simply an oblique section of the aorta which is unrolled and sinuous, as is common in elderly patients.

This is a very peculiar image of calcification of both suprarenal glands, clearly suggesting a chronic process. This may be the result of:
– Infection, e.g., tuberculosis
– Suprarenal hemorrhage

Scan 82 (section level 2, p. 96) shows calcified suprarenal hematomas (26).

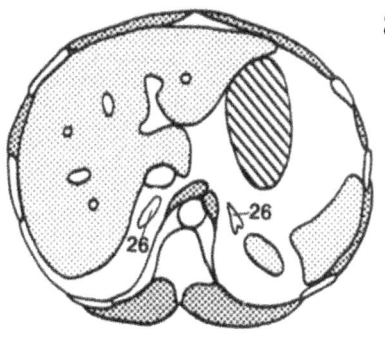

In spite of their wide differences these eight images bear in common that each patient has Conn's syndrome, with primary hyperaldosteronism and nonexistent plasmatic renin activity. When faced with such a context, CT is the first technique to be used in the search for the cause of this affliction. This is either adenoma or hyperplasia.

Adenoma is found in 80% of cases. There is a typical rounded mass of less than 2 cm diameter, hanging on one of the branches of the suprarenal gland. It is unilateral and has a low density due to its fatty content.

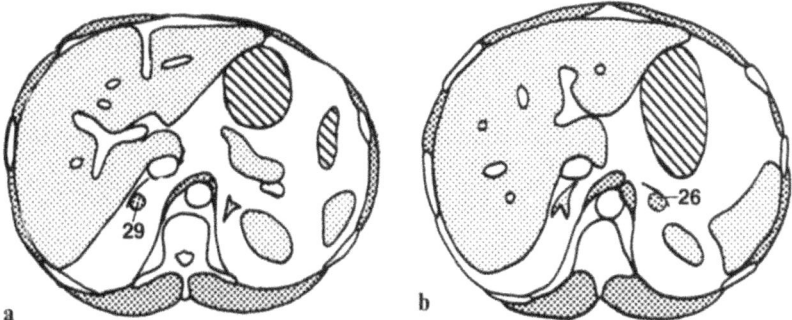

a (section level 3, p. 97): A right suprarenal adenoma (29).
b (section level 2, p. 96): A left suprarenal adenoma (26).

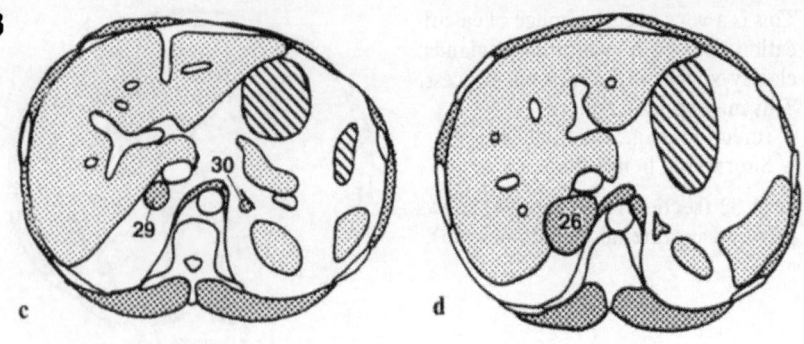

c   d

But there are exceptions:
c (section level 3, p. 97): Bilateral adenoma (*29, 30*), **d** (section level 2, p. 96):
Adenoma of large size (*26*).

Bilateral hyperplasia occurs in 20% of cases and, unlike adenoma, cannot be
treated by surgery. A thickness of more than 10 mm in the branches of the
suprarenal gland confirms the diagnosis. Four further scans were made to
investigate both suprarenal beds in one patient.

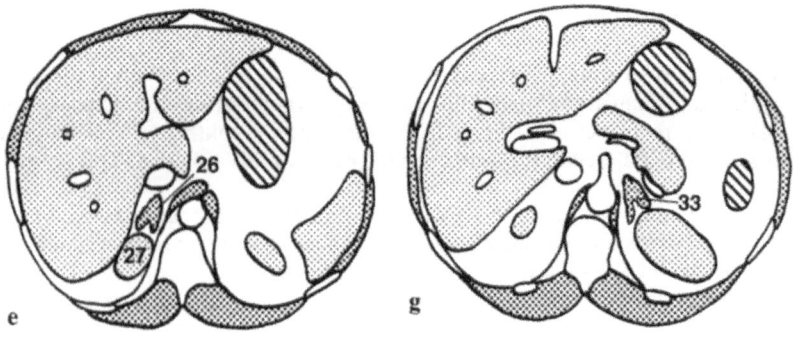

e   g

e, f (section level 2, p. 96): The hypertrophic suprarenal gland (*26*) situated
anterior to the upper pole of the right kidney (*27*).

g, h (section level 4, p. 98): The left suprarenal gland (*33*) has an increased
volume, but its form is unchanged as compared with that of the right one. This is
characteristic for hyperplasia.

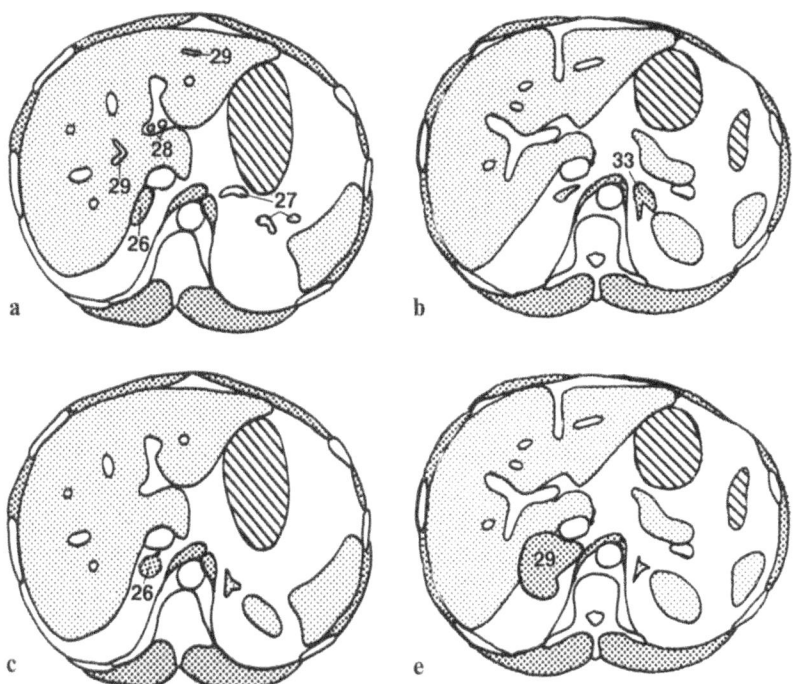

Two anomalies are striking in this series of scans 84 a–f.
- The suprarenals are pathologic
- The abundance of abdominal fat

They nevertheless suggest a common diagnosis: Cushing's syndrome.

a, b: Bilateral hyperplasia (*13, 18*) of the suprarenal glands. This is the most common aspect (80%).

 a (section level 2, p. 96): This scan performed during bolus injection shows, besides the hypertrophic suprarenal gland (*26*), the heterogeneous enhancement of the spleen (see also scan 57), the opacification of loops of the splenic artery (*27*), of the hepatic artery (*28*), and of the intraparenchymatous branches (*29*) of the latter.

 b (section level 4, p. 98): This section is taken 3 cm below the previous one; it confirms the bilaterality of the hyperplasia by demonstrating the hypertrophic left suprarenal gland (*33*).

 c, d (section level 2, p. 96): The suprarenal adenoma (*26*) is second in order of frequency (15%). Its densities, like those of hyperplasia, are often low (−5 to +30 HU) because its composition is strongly adipose.

 e, f (section level 3, p. 97): The least frequent etiology (5%) is the carcinoma (*29*), which is often voluminous and necrotic, invading the liver, as shown here (*4*).

 In all cases abundant fat facilitates the investigation and orientates the diagnosis.

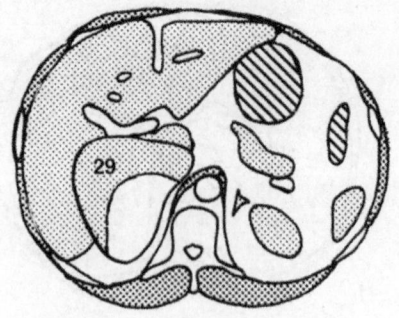

One notes here a voluminous, calcified, suprarenal mass on the right. Discussion of its origin must consider the following possibilities:

Infectious cause	tuberculosis (see scan 80)
	histoplasmosis
	hydatidosis
Tumoral cause	sympathoblastoma
	secreting or nonsecreting carcinoma
	Cushing's adenoma (nonfunctional Conn's adenomas calcify rarely)

Scan 85 (section level 3, p. 97). The calcified mass (*29*) in this case is a sign of a nonsecreting adenoma.

Subject Index